32.50

369 0166869

KU-407-161

THE CASE-CONTROL METHOD

MONOGRAPHS IN EPIDEMIOLOGY AND BIOSTATISTICS

Edited by Albert Hofman, Michael Marmot, Jonathan Samet, David Z. Savitz

THE CASE-CONTROL METHOD

DESIGN AND APPLICATIONS

Haroutune K. Armenian, MD, DrPH

President, American University of Armenia
Yerevan, Armenia
Professor Emeritus
Bloomberg School of Public Health
The Johns Hopkins University
Baltimore, Maryland
Professor in Residence School of Public Health
University of California, Los Angeles
Los Angeles, California

OXFORD
UNIVERSITY PRESS

2009

OXFORD
UNIVERSITY PRESS

Oxford University Press, Inc., publishes works that further
Oxford University's objective of excellence
in research, scholarship, and education.

Oxford New York
Auckland Cape Town Dar es Salaam Hong Kong Karachi
Kuala Lumpur Madrid Melbourne Mexico City Nairobi
New Delhi Shanghai Taipei Toronto

With offices in
Argentina Austria Brazil Chile Czech Republic France Greece
Guatemala Hungary Italy Japan Poland Portugal Singapore
South Korea Switzerland Thailand Turkey Ukraine Vietnam

Published by Oxford University Press, Inc.
198 Madison Avenue, New York, New York 10016
www.oup.com

Oxford is a registered trademark of Oxford University Press

Library of Congress Cataloging-in-Publication Data

Armenian, Haroutune K.
The case-control method : design and applications / Haroutune Armenian.
p. ; cm.
Includes bibliographical references.
ISBN 978-0-19-518711-3
1. Case-control method. I. Title.
[DNLM: 1. Case-Control Studies. WA 950 A728c 2009]
RA652.2.M3A76 2009
610.72—dc22
2008041127

9 8 7 6 5 4 3 2 1
Printed in the United States of America
on acid-free paper

To my parents Krikor and Arshaluys Armenian
for guiding us to avoid becoming cases
without strict controls

PREFACE

Epidemiology has evolved into a discipline with a multitude of applications. A variety of public health and health services problems are investigated using epidemiologic methods. The complexity of some of these problems has fragmented the field into a number of subspecialties and today it is not uncommon to read about "epidemiologies." The epidemiologic methods and a common system of inferences are what maintain the discipline as a unified whole.

The case-control method (and, to a lesser extent, its case-based variants) has become a most important tool in the armamentarium of today's investigator of health problems. Over the past 50 years, this method has been tested in numerous investigations. Also over this period of time, the method has been refined, solutions have been found to some of the problems plaguing it, and its investigative approaches have been systematized.

This book was made possible by 18 years of teaching a course on the case-control method to a large number of students from a variety of backgrounds at the Department of Epidemiology of the Bloomberg School of Public Health of the Johns Hopkins University. As a text it will help its users to address a number of general and specific questions dealing with the case-control and other case-based methods. Included in these questions are:

- How to design and implement a case-control study that minimizes biases?
- How to interpret data and present the results from a case-control study?
- How to use the method in a variety of problem-solving situations?

The starting point for a case-control study is the problem at hand. Most of the time the problem is an undesirable health outcome. An initial study of a case with such an outcome can provide a wealth of information and can help us develop hypotheses about the determinants of the outcome. As we start developing our case-control study, we may benefit from a review of a series of cases. An assessment of the common threads between such cases helps further refine our hypotheses and improve our definition of case status. Hence, the first chapter of this book deals with an exposition of the methods, the inferential limitations but also the potential uses of case investigation, and a study of a series of cases. In order not to overstate the argument for these approaches, this first chapter provides a short historical overview of the development of the comparative method where a group of controls makes our inferences more meaningful. The second chapter is an overview of the case-control method and our approach to inferences using this method. Chapter 3 deals with the most important steps in the design of a case-control study, including selection of cases and controls and measurement of exposure. Approaches that avoid biases characterize this chapter and Chapter 4. The chapter on Alternative Case-Based Designs (Chapter 5) presents the newer methods of case-cohort and case-crossover studies with their strengths and limitations. The next chapter (Chapter 6) of the book deals with analytic methods. Starting with standard steps in the analysis of case-control studies, this chapter presents bivariate and multivariate methods for both unmatched and matched study designs. The final section of the book (starting from Chapter 7) provides a wealth of applications of the case-control and case-based methods in five chapters, including outbreak investigation, genetic epidemiology, evaluation of interventions, and evaluation of screening programs.

This book has a much stronger emphasis on uses and applications of the case-control and case-based methods than on statistical methods. Two previously published excellent texts on the case-control method by Schelesselman and by Breslow and Day present a more statistical approach. Both of these texts helped define and standardize the case-control method and its analysis. Today, we are exposed to several good statistical analytic methods that continue to evolve and change. These methods are extensively available in standard statistical software packages and accessible to most users of this text. The use and understanding of this current text requires familiarity with an introductory level of epidemiology and biostatistics only.

This is a book for the epidemiologist as well as for the occasional user of the case-control and other case-based methods. It is a treatise that helps one to design a good case-control study but also to critically evaluate such a study using a step-by-step approach.

Acknowledgments: Charlotte Gerczak, Mary Rybczynski, and Eric Seaberg.

CONTENTS

Contributors

Haroutune K. Armenian,
MD, DrPH
*President, American University
of Armenia
Yerevan, Armenia
Professor Emeritus
Bloomberg School of Public Health
The Johns Hopkins University
Baltimore, Maryland
Professor in Residence School of
Public Health
University of California,
Los Angeles
Los Angeles, California*

M. Daniele Fallin, PhD
*Associate Professor
Department of Epidemiology
Bloomberg School of Public Health
The Johns Hopkins University
Baltimore, Maryland*

W. H. Linda Kao, PhD, MHS
*Associate Professor
Department of Epidemiology
Bloomberg School of Public Health
The Johns Hopkins University
Baltimore, Maryland*

Miriam Khlat, PhD
*Senior Researcher
Institut National d'Etudes
Démographiques (INED)
Paris, France*

Gayane Yenokyan, MD, MPH
*Doctoral Candidate, Epidemiology
Bloomberg School of Public Health
The Johns Hopkins University
Baltimore, Maryland*

THE CASE-CONTROL METHOD

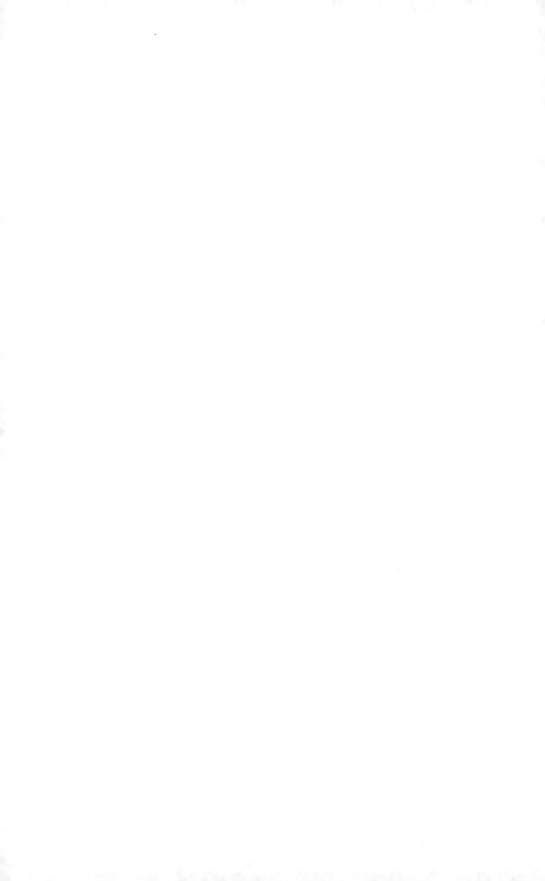

1

FROM CASE INVESTIGATION TO THE CASE-CONTROL METHOD: INFORMATION FOR DECISION MAKING

Haroutune K. Armenian

OUTLINE

This chapter aims to

1. explain the role of epidemiology as an information science;
2. explain the strengths and limitations of case investigation and a study of a series of cases in assessing a health problem and helping develop hypotheses; and
3. provide landmarks in the history of the case-control method.

1.1 EPIDEMIOLOGY AS AN INFORMATION SCIENCE

Like other scientific disciplines entrenched within a professional practice environment, *epidemiology is an information science*. It aims to influence *decision making* in a number of situations. Data generated in epidemiology is used as information—albeit in a transformed format—for making decisions by individuals, health professionals, and policy makers in dealing with various problems.

When a new epidemiological finding of an association between exposure to a product and a cancer is announced, it causes concern to the users of the product who hear about it (*information*) and who will consider discontinuing the use of the product (*possible decision*). The health professionals who also read or hear about this announcement will try to become better informed but may also advise patients and others to avoid the exposure until further information is made available. Similarly, the policy maker will ask for further elucidation prior to making a decision as to whether something needs to be done at this time on the policy level about this exposure.

Epidemiology is also *purposive*. Its methods and knowledge are to be used for the ultimate purpose of *prevention of disease, disability, and death*. Although, this may sound like a very pragmatic interpretation of the role of epidemiology, it helps us visualize the discipline in the context of problem solving for public health and medicine. Whether we are dealing with a research finding or a surveillance report, we are interested in their ultimate significance as to how they would influence health and disease in the community.

Because of such an important public role, epidemiology is under *constant public scrutiny*. Epidemiologists have a level of social responsibility that is comparable to other public service professions. Decisions on the relevance of epidemiologic findings are influenced by such a public role. Prior to recommending a certain course of action following an outbreak of salmonellosis, it is important that we have the data that support our proposed course of action "beyond reasonable doubt." Epidemiology and epidemiologists have been chastised in the past by the media and the public for rushing to conclusions when the data did not provide the full spectrum of evidence.

Thus, the data that forms the basis for the information–decision continuum needs to be very well scrutinized as to its validity and reliability. While carrying out investigations of health problems, appropriate epidemiologic methods help us

1. minimize *systematic errors or bias*,
2. explore the presence of alternative explanations to our observations by controlling the effect of *confounders*, and
3. assess potential *interactions*.

Epidemiology also provides us with approaches to interpret and understand the significance of our findings, as well as ways to improve the information value of our observations.

> Box 1.1 Determinants of the Value
> of Information
>
> • Validity
> • Utility
> • Generalizability
> • Timeliness
> • Distribution
> • Quantity
> • Cost

The *value of information* is a function of its *validity*, its *utility* to multiple users, its ability to be used in multiple situations (*generalizability*), *timeliness* with which it is provided, its *distribution*, its *amount*, and the *cost* of producing it (see Box 1.1).

The first of these characteristics of information is its *validity*. Validity is measured by sensitivity and specificity. How good is the data in presenting a true picture of the reality or the situation that we are assessing? In a situation where we do not have data at a high level of sensitivity and/or specificity, we may be reluctant to ascribe any significant value to the findings of the study.

Utility, distribution, and generalizability are other characteristics of information that improve the value of the data. The more users and the broader representation of these users, the greater the value we get from our data.

Timeliness of the information is a critical characteristic of data. A delayed data provision is not effectively used for decision making. The *amount*, and the *cost* of producing the data influence our judgment of the value of the information.

As illustrated in the Figure below, we use epidemiologic methods to generate information that undergoes a process of inferences for decision making and hopefully for action-intervention.

Information Generation → Decision Process → Action
Epidemiologic Methods → Process of Inferences → Intervention

The above-described concepts of epidemiology as an information science are applicable to the breadth of our methods including the case-control and other case-based methods.

From the individual patient to major endemics, we deal with a spectrum of issues that need to be addressed and investigated. Thus, the unit of observation for our investigations as well as the sampling strategies of our study population is very much dictated by the problem under consideration.

There is a continuum from case investigation and case series to more complex case-based designs such as case-control or case-crossover studies. In a clinical environment, the investigation of a disease starts at the level of the individual case or case series. At such a stage, problems are defined and a number of alternative hypotheses generated about the case or the series of cases. The move from case series to the case-control approach is warranted when these hypotheses need to be explored and tested.

Recently, in a review of the "Origins and early development of the case-control study," Paneth et al. (1) trace these origins to the realm of patient care. According to these authors, there are concepts and practices in a clinical context that underlie the development of the case-control method. These include *caseness* of a specific disease and interest in explaining *etiology* at the individual level; the practice of *anamnesis*, or taking a history from the patient, and grouping cases into *series*; and comparing groups of patients to elicit differences. Our discussion of the evolution from case investigation to controlled comparisons follows a similar appreciation of these origins.

1.2 CASE INVESTIGATION

1.2.1 *Questions at the Clinical Level*

A number of questions underlie the investigation of a single individual with an illness or other health problem at the clinical level. These include

- What is the problem?
- Why this case?
- How can we manage this case?
- What will be the long-term consequences of the disease and its management?
- What can we learn from this case that will help us understand and manage similar situations?

The last question is an attempt to generalize from this individual patient and is also of epidemiological interest. As an epidemiologist-clinician, Professor Roy Acheson encouraged medical students to consider the following question during their investigation of patients: "Why did this patient get this disease at this time?" (2).

As a result of our investigation of a case, we can address most of these questions and make decisions about the types of action we need to take. Also, we generate valuable data about the etiology of this case that

Table 1.1. Uses of the Case Investigation Method

- Etiologic Research
- Pathology Investigation
- Clinical Case Investigation
- Medicolegal Product Liability Cases
- Genetics
- Occupational Medicine
- Medical Social Work
- Administration

may be useful for future prevention of similar cases. Hannah et al. investigated a case of Creutzfeld-Jakob disease (CJD) as to possible cause of transmission of this chronic encephalopathy. The patient had received a graft of dural matter during a neurosurgical operation. The donor of the graft had also later developed neurological signs and symptoms. The findings in this case dictate that we establish more rigorous controls in selecting our donors in such operations (3).

Most case investigations are conducted to address the problems presented by a single patient at the clinical level. For most of these it is important for the health professionals conducting the investigation to understand and explain the patient's problem in order to prescribe the proper treatment regimen. When we are dealing with individuals, we need to be able to "privatize risk," to assess the individual's risk and inform the individual about it. Most preventive action depends on decisions by individuals. Improving the tools for predicting risk at the level of the individual may assist in more effective preventive action.

Table 1.1 provides a list of uses of the case investigation in the clinical and public health environment.

1.2.2 An Epidemiological Tool

Many a time our understanding of risk at the group level may not be directly applicable at the individual level (4). Thus, the refinement of case investigation as an epidemiologic tool takes on an added significance.

In epidemiology, and as a method of exploring health problems, case investigation provides an in-depth study of a single person and the facts and events surrounding that person. The methods used in case investigation allow integration and synthesis of data; involve a targeted approach in addressing the health problems, and use methods from a variety of disciplines.

From a broad descriptive and clinical concern, the case investigation is useful for general exploratory studies, as well as explanatory for individual cases. In epidemiology a case investigation is useful to investigate a rare disease situation whether limited or defined by geography or uncommon pathology. Sometimes the pathology is very common but there are epidemiologic features that are unusual. For example, although a particular type of malignancy like cancer of the colon or prostate may be quite common in later years, such a condition in a person under 20 years of age is very unusual and needs to be investigated to explain its occurrence.

1.2.3 At the Health Department

Case investigation is used in health departments for investigating cases of conditions identified through surveillance and monitoring programs. For example, in a region where its incidence is very low, a case of typhoid fever that is reported to the health department is investigated systematically to explain the underlying mode of transmission in this particular person. The purpose behind such an investigation is to try to prevent further cases of the disease. Also, at the health department, a case of active tuberculosis or sexually transmitted disease is studied through an investigation of contacts to assess the manner in which the infection was transmitted and to try to prevent the spread of the infection among contacts.

One of the advantages of case investigation is that usually both the patient and the physician have a higher motivation to participate in the investigation than in a case-control study since the results of the investigation may be of immediate benefit to the patient (5).

Thus, case investigation is useful in epidemiology, to

- develop a high *index of suspicion*. If our observations can form the basis of a reasonable hypothesis, case investigation may help us prevent further cases of the particular condition in the future on the basis of "reasonable concern."
- study *rare conditions* in a situation where we have serious limitations of power for a larger-scale study;
- understand the condition in more detail for some *clues to etiology*. In evaluating potential etiological relationships, the case investigation allows us to gather good information about some of the judgment criteria such as time sequence and biological plausibility, as well as consistency of the observation across similar cases.
- investigate the *epidemiologically odd or unusual cases* of disease in a geographically isolated situation and/or in a small number of cases within a limited population base.

1.3 STUDIES OF CASE SERIES

A study of a case series is one of the most commonly used tools of clinical investigation. In many specific examples, a case series was the first study that brought forth a new hypothesis and tested a number of ideas. In 1981, the first report of a small number of young homosexual men with unusual disorders of Kaposi's sarcoma and Pneumocystis pneumonia led to the recognition of the massive epidemic of AIDS and helped develop initial hypotheses about its etiology (6).

A study of a case series tries to address a number of questions including the following:

- Are there any group or common characteristics that can be identified for the cases of this condition?
- Does the management of these cases follow established standards?
- Are there any subgroups of people with this condition that need special attention?
- What are the geographic distribution and the time trends of these cases?

Case series are reviewed in a number of situations:

Clinical research. Here the investigator is primarily interested in characterizing the condition for diagnostic purposes, evaluating various treatment alternatives that are being used in the community, and predicting prognosis in people with the condition. La Grenade et al. studied a case series of infective dermatitis (ID) in children and compared their cases with patients with atopic dermatitis to characterize better ID. They described a number of clinical and laboratory differences that characterize ID (7).

Outbreak investigation. In most outbreak investigations, the initial phase starts with a review of the known or identified cases of the disease. The investigator uses the series of initial cases to identify some common patterns of the people with the disease to be used to develop an "epidemiologic definition" of cases and to formulate some preliminary hypotheses. For example, through such a review one may identify that the majority of the cases belong to a certain ethnic group or belong to a club that has just had its annual dinner party. Pollanen et al. described a cluster of a series of eight cases of sudden unexplained death in Asian immigrants in Metropolitan Toronto. Their investigation did not reveal any specific factors that were common to all these cases except for their Asian immigrant status (8).

Evaluative programs. One may be able to assess program impact by reviewing a series of cases and their management. A more specific type of evaluation using the case series is done for quality assurance purposes. The management of a series of cases is compared to some expected external standards of care. Good compliance with external professional guidelines of management can be accepted as a sign of good quality of care.

Genetic research. Recently genetic investigations have used a case only series approach for making inferences about etiology. This will be further elaborated in Chapter 8.

Ethnographic research. A study of a series of cases of a certain condition is a very useful tool to find out different aspects of the anthropology of the condition in a community. What are some dominant perceptions about the etiology of the condition? How does the disease or condition affect the life of the individual, the family, and the community? What is the standard management of this condition in this community? What is the historical perspective on the prognosis and long-term effects of the condition? These are the type of questions that can be addressed from an in-depth ethnographic study of a series of cases of the disease.

The major problem with an investigation of a case series is our limited ability to make inferences because of the absence of a control or comparison group. As stated by Philip Cole " a case series is an aborted case-control study; there is no control group but there may be some basis for suggesting that cases have an unusual frequency of exposure to some presumptive cause of the disease" (9). If we observe in a case series that a vast majority of the cases are exposed to a certain agent, one can not state that this finding characterizes the condition, unless we rule out in a control group of people without the condition that that there is no such elevated exposure. Bailar et al. (10) reviewed 20 clinical studies of medical treatment with no internal controls. They proposed a set of actions that will add strength to such studies. These include *specifying a hypothesis* before the results are observed, *planning the analysis* before the data are generated, and having reasonable grounds at the outset that the results can be *generalizable to others* with the condition. One can also use these features when assessing the validity of a series of cases

Another problem with a number of case series is that these studies are usually conducted in tertiary medical care facilities, and because of selection, the study may be limited to the more severe forms of the condition. Hence, what we observe about the condition from these case series may not be generalizable to the breadth of people with that condition.

Often in a case series all patients are coming from the same hospital or practice (11).

To help with inferences, many case series may use data from the same community about the frequency of the exposure in the general population. Thus, if the proportion of smokers in our case series is 40%, then this figure can be compared with data from other sources in the same community, such as from an unrelated survey. The data from the community will act as a yardstick against which the 40% exposure rate is compared. In a study on obesity, smoking, and psoriasis, Herron et al. (12) compared a series of patients with psoriasis as to obesity and smoking with data from the Behavioral Surveillance System of the Utah population. Compared to the survey of the Utah population, cases of psoriasis had a higher prevalence of obesity and smoking.

One of the problems that affect both case investigation and case series is the analysis of data from small numbers of cases. Bayesian analysis may provide us with a tool to make the appropriate inferences in such situations where we are dealing with small numbers (5).

There are a number of approaches that can help us develop a hypothesis. These include

1. an assessment of the magnitude and distribution of a public health problem and the issues related to its prevention and control;
2. clinical observations in a case investigation or case series;
3. observations from experimental animal and human studies;
4. a review of previous investigations of the problem in the literature;
5. formal and informal scientific meetings;
6. a systematic review of the evidence.

In developing and stating a hypothesis one needs to formulate the question in a manner that specifies clearly the

- outcome of interest;
- determinant(s) of the outcome;
- direction of the effect of determinant to outcome.

1.4 A HISTORICAL REVIEW OF CONTROLLED COMPARISONS

1.4.1 Overview

The development of controlled comparisons is one of the most prominent forces of change that we have seen over the past two centuries in medicine and public health. Controlled comparisons are used to identify etiology, to define disease and its appropriate diagnostic classification, and to assess the efficacy and effectiveness of therapy and interventions. Controlled comparisons have been used to improve the strength of the argument in all three of these situations.

One of the earliest persons to use the controlled comparisons in medicine and public health was the French professor Pierre Charles Alexandre Louis (13). He lived early in the 19th century during the reign of Napoleon Bonaparte and used the comparative approach to make judgments about the effectiveness of established therapies of his day. He is remembered as the person who challenged the rationale of a number of treatments in the medical armamentarium of the day. The following is a quote from his writings:

In any epidemic, for instance, let us suppose five hundred of the sick, taken indiscriminately, to be subjected to one kind of treatment, and five hundred others, taken in the same manner, to be treated in a different mode; if the mortality is greater among the first than among the second, must we not conclude that the treatment was less appropriate, or less efficacious in the first class, than in the second? (P.C.A. Louis; 13)

In his treatise on tuberculosis, Louis proposed to make judgment on the possible hereditary nature of the disease by comparing the occurrence of tuberculosis in the parents of patients with the disease to a sample from the general population (1).

According to the Lilienfelds, Louis, through a number of followers and students influenced the development of epidemiology and public health as scientific disciplines (13). One of his American students was Elisha Bartlett. The following quote is from the writings of Bartlett:

There should be no selection of cases.
There is one sense in which knowledge of the normal structure and the physiological actions of the body may be said to be necessary for knowledge of its abnormal structure and its pathological actions. We need the former as a *standard of comparison* for the latter.

In the second half of the 19th century, the successes of the bacteriological revolution led by Pasteur and Koch dampened the development of the observational comparative method in epidemiology. The laboratory-based experimental approach became the predominant scientific investigative mode and the Henle-Koch postulates set the rules and the standards for assessing etiology. To define etiological relationships one needed (1) to find the etiologic agent in every case of the disease; (2) not to detect the agent in people without the disease; and (3) to successfully transmit the disease through the agent. If these conditions were satisfied then the relationship between the agent and the disease was causal.

An example of this approach to the etiology of disease is illustrated by the work of Harry Graham in 1900, in Beirut. In a series of experiments, Graham was able to demonstrate that dengue fever was transmitted through the mosquito bite. Unfortunately, he identified the wrong mosquito. In the first of his experiments a nursing mother who was taken ill with the dengue fever was allowed to sleep in the same room as the infant she continued nursing but each of the rooms she used was always cleared from mosquitoes using chlorine gas. In the absence of the mosquito the disease was not transmitted to the infant or during similar other experiments to others in this epidemic of dengue (14).

The first two decades of the 20th century were marked by developments that eventually led to new thinking regarding the germ theory of the bacteriologic era. Using essentially statistical and demographic analysis of data, Goldberger (1916) was able to uphold a nutritional cause for the etiology of pellagra (15). It was about this time that F. Stuart Chapin (1917) promoted the "experimental" method in sociology (16). One of the disciples of Chapin, Stuart Carter Dodd, an associate professor of sociology at the American University of Beirut, was interested in health problems as social phenomena and conducted a controlled experiment on rural hygiene in Syria. He published his results in 1934 (17,18).

The experiment he set up was to test whether the introduction of a hygienic culture in two Syrian villages would affect the health of the people. Following baseline examinations in both villages, Dodd and his colleagues introduced health education in one village and no intervention in the other village. Two years following the baseline examination they could not observe any differences between the two groups as to health status. His interpretation for this lack of effect in the experimental group was that of diffusion. Since the two villages were not too far apart, the hygienic culture had diffused from the experimental to the control village.

In 1920, Broders conducted one of the earliest known case-control studies (19). He compared 537 cases of squamous-cell epithelioma of the lip and 500 controls without the condition. In 1926, Lane-Clayton conducted the first case-control study assessing the etiology of breast cancer (20). Other early case-control studies include Pearl's study of tuberculosis and cancer (21), and the study of etiologic factors of carcinoma of the penis by Schrek and Lenowitz in 1947 (22). For the first time, these latter authors compared several control groups to their cases.

In 1949–50, four case-control studies appeared in the literature describing the association of cigarette smoking and lung cancer.

Considering the well-established habit of smoking at the time, including among the most prominent scientists, these papers generated a great deal of controversy and discussion, much of which was directed against the relatively new method of case-control studies. As a result of the ensuing intense discussion involving epidemiologists and biostatisticians, the weaknesses of the case-control method were identified and appropriate solutions found to these problems. In a way the story of cigarette smoking and lung cancer is the story of the development of the case-control method. Of these four case-control studies, the story of the study by Morton Levin et al. will be presented here (23, 24).

Born in Tbilisi, Georgia, Morton Levin was a physician who graduated with a DrPH in epidemiology from Johns Hopkins School of Hygiene and Public Health. Wade Hampton Frost was his mentor. Following graduation from Hopkins in 1936, he was invited to the Roswell Park Memorial Institute for cancer research to be engaged in research on the potential infectious origin of cancer.

In 1938, admissions office personnel at Roswell Park asked Levin to review the admission questionnaire that all patients were asked to complete. Morton Levin, with a hunch about the potential role of cigarette smoking in cancer, added a couple of questions about smoking to the admissions questionnaire. About a decade later he revisited the admissions questionnaire data on smoking in a nested case-control study about lung cancer. He compared cases of lung cancer to four control groups (24). His study was free of interviewer and other biases that plagued other case-control studies on the subject. Since information about smoking was collected prior to the establishment of a diagnosis and through a process of data collection that was independent of case and control identification, his findings were probably more credible.

A number of landmarks in the development of the case-control method occurred between the 1950s and 1960s, including the calculation of the odds ratio by Cornfield (25), the assessment of confounding and interaction, and the description of a host of biases that could plague these studies. The development of the Mantel–Haenzel chi squared summary statistic pooled estimator of relative risk in 1959 paved the way to controlling confounding and multivariate analyses (26). Box 1.2 lists some of the names used over the years to refer to the case control method.

1.4.2 What Do We Learn from History?

A review of historical developments in epidemiology helps us understand the forces and events behind the development of new knowledge and also

```
Box 1.2 Nomenclature

Case-control
Case-referrent
Compeer
Retrospective
Case-history
(Trohoc)
```

new methodologies like the case-control method. Through the last two centuries, new problems in public health and medicine have provided the impetus for the development of new methodologies and have thus invigorated the discipline and enriched the tools in our armamentarium.

Uncertainty in therapeutics highlighted the need for inferences based on measurement and Louis developed the comparative approach in response. Major epidemics led to the formulation of social epidemiologic concepts and field-based methods by Snow, as well as in the initiation of the laboratory-based experimental method of Pasteur and Koch. Early in the 20th century epidemiologists who were investigating such chronic conditions as pellagra, tuberculosis, and cancer had to incorporate a more sophisticated approach to measurement and statistical reasoning. Some of the sociometric methods that were being developed at the time were introduced into disease etiological studies.

With the case-control method epidemiologists had a powerful tool that could be used effectively to address the investigative needs of a large number of health problems that were awaiting attention.

REFERENCES

1. Paneth N, Susser E, Susser M. Origins and early development of the case-control study. In: Morabia A. ed. *A History of Epidemiologic Methods and Concepts*. Basel/Switzerland: Birkhauser Verlag; 2004:291-311.
2. Rose G. Sick individuals and sick populations. *Int J Epidemiol*. 1985;14:32-38.
3. Hannah EL, Belay ED, Gambetti P, et al. Transmissible spongiform encephalopathies; prion disease. *Neurology*. 2001;56:1080-1083.
4. Rockhill B. The privatization of risk. *Am J Public Health*. 2001;91:365-368.
5. Dunson DB. Commentary: practical advantages of Bayesian analysis of epidemiologic data. *Am J Epidemiol*. 2001;153:1222-1226.
6. Durack DT. Opportunistic infections and Kaposi's sarcoma in homosexual men. *N Engl J Med*. 1981;305:1465-1467.
7. La Grenade L, Manns A, Fletcher V, et al. Clinical, pathologic, and immunologic features of Human T-Lymphotrophic virus Type I-Associated infective dermatitis in children. *Arch Dermatol*. 1998;134:439-444.

8. Pollanen MS, Chiasson DA, Cairns J, Young JG. Sudden unexplained death in Asian immigrants: recognition of a syndrome in Metropolitan Toronto. *Can Med Assoc J.* 1996;155:537-540.

9. Cole P. The evolving case-control study. *J Chron Dis.* 1979;32:15-27.

10. Bailar JC 3rd, Louis TA, Lavori PW, Polansky M. Studies without internal controls. *N Engl J Med.* 1984;311:156-162.

11. Grisso JA. Making comparisons. *The Lancet.* 1993;342:157-160.

12. Herron MD, Hinckley M, Hoffman MS, et al. Impact of obesity and smoking on psoriasis presentation and management. *Arch Dermatol.* 2005;141:1527-1534.

13. Lilienfeld A, Lilienfeld D. A century of case-control studies: progress? *J Chronic Dis.* 1979;32:5-13.

14. Graham H. The dengue: a study of its pathology and mode of propagation. *J Tropical Med.* 1903;6:209-214.

15. Goldberger J. The transmissibility of Pellagra. Experimental attempts at transmission to the human subject. *Public Health Reports.* 1916;31:3159-3173.

16. Chapin FS. The experimental method and sociology. *The Scientific Monthly.* 1917;February:133-144.

17. Dodd SC. *A Controlled Experiment on Rural Hygiene in Syria.* American University of Beirut, Social Sciences Series 1934; No. 7:336-463.

18. Breslow NE, Day NE. *Statistical Methods in Cancer Research*, Volume 1—*The analysis of case-control studies.* Lyon: International Agency for Research on Cancer; 1980.

19. Broders AC. Squamous-cell epithelioma of the lip. A study of five hundred and thirty-seven cases. *JAMA.* 1920;74:656-664.

20. Lane-Claypon JE. *A further report on cancer of the breast, with special reference to its associated antecedent conditions.* Ministry of Health reports on public health and medical subjects, No. 32. London: HMSO; 1926.

21. Pearl R. Cancer and tuberculosis. *American Journal of Hygiene.* 1929;9:97-159.

22. Schrek R, Lenowitz H. Etiological factors in carcinoma of. the penis. *Cancer Research.* 1947;7:180-187.

23. Thun MJ. When truth is unwelcome: the first reports on smoking and lung cancer. *Bull WHO.* 2005;83:144-145.

24. Levin ML, Goldstein H, Gerhardt PR. Cancer and tobacco smoking. A preliminary report. *JAMA.* 1950;143:336-338.

25. Cornfield J. A method of estimating comparative rates from clinical data. Application to cancer of the lung, breast and cervix. *J Natl Can Inst.* 1951;11:1269-1275.

26. Mantel N, Haenszel W. Statistical aspects of the analysis of data from retrospective studies of disease. *J Natl Cancer Inst.* 1959;22:719-48.

2

PROBLEM INVESTIGATION AND INFERENCES USING THE CASE-CONTROL METHOD

Haroutune K. Armenian

OUTLINE

This chapter aims to

1. explain why the case-control method is a problem-solving tool;
2. describe some of the limitations of the case-control method;
3. identify situations where the use of the case-control method is indicated;
4. discuss the options for making inferences from case-control studies; and
5. describe an approach for evaluating case-control studies.

2.1 PROBLEMS THAT CAN BE INVESTIGATED

Almost all problems that need to be investigated in public health and medicine would benefit from the use of the case-control method, provided it is used appropriately.

Currently, the major uses of the method can be grouped under three headings:

Etiologic research. This is where traditionally much of the methodology of the case-control studies was developed. *What causes the disease?* This question stems from both a scientific interest and from our concern for prevention. If we want to prevent a disease then we need to know its causes. From identifying the causes of lung cancer to revealing risk factors for abdominal aneurysms, the case-control method has been a very effective investigative tool in tracing etiology. In a clinical investigation of the role of Epstein-Barr virus (EBV) in the etiology of daily persistent headaches, Diaz-Mitoma et al. (1) compared 32 cases of the condition to 32 age-matched healthy volunteer controls. Using EBV excretion and/or early antigen titers as their indication of "active" infection with EBV, they reported that 84% of the patients with new daily persistent headaches and 25% of the controls had such evidence of infection. Although such studies may be marred with a number of methodological problems, they are frequently used to make inferences about what differentiates people with the disease from those without.

Acute event investigation. In the practice of public health and epidemiology, we are faced with a number of situations where we need to carry on an investigation within a short time frame to expedite decision making and intervention. *How to deal with a major problem at hand?* Acute events such as an outbreak or epidemic, or a disaster that affects the community sometimes overwhelm the health services and professionals. During these events the health services need to cope with multiple demands and pressures. Epidemiology provides the tools to assess such situations but also to investigate the problems to address them through a rational decision-making process. The case-control method has been used extensively over the past 30 years to investigate such acute events (Chapter 7).

Evaluation. A number of programs and new treatments are initiated every month to address the needs of the community and those people who are sick. Because we are dealing with limited resources in the health services, it is important to assess the effectiveness of our interventions and our programs. *How well are we doing?* This is a question that is part of the rational management of any project or program. Accountability to an organization or to the general public is part of our social responsibility as health professionals. The case-control method can be a powerful tool for evaluating programs and other interventions (Chapter 9).

The common thread for all these uses of the case-control method is the fact that by using this approach we are addressing the problem at hand in a relatively expeditious manner. In doing so, we are hastening preventive action that hopefully will improve situations in the future.

Geoffrey Rose defines two major directions for public health action: *prevention by the high risk strategy* where individuals who are at high risk for the disease are identified and managed like in a screening program, or *prevention through the population strategy*. "The whole basis of the case-control is to discover how sick and healthy individuals differ" (2). In the latter approach the preventive program will identify interventions that involve the whole population and may be more effective in preventing a higher proportion of illness. Rose defines the pros and cons of each of these approaches. As presented in Chapter 1, case investigation and case series have a focus on sick individuals and will help primarily a high-risk strategy of prevention, while the case-control method aims to learn about the causes of incidence and to tackle etiology in our broader population-based preventive effort.

2.2 DEFINITIONS OF CASE-CONTROL STUDIES

Table 2.1 lists a number of definitions for the case-control method.

Essentially the case-control design is a comparison of a group of persons with a certain outcome or condition with another group of

Table 2.1. Definitions of the Case-Control Method

The retrospective method determines the attributes, or the risk factors, associated with a particular disease, by contrasting a series of patients with the disease with a control group who do not have the disease. Philip Sartwell (3)

A case-control study is an investigation into the extent to which persons selected because they have a specific disease (the cases) and comparable persons who do not have the disease (the controls) have been exposed to the disease's possible risk factors in order to evaluate the hypothesis that one or more of these is a cause of the disease. Philip Cole (4)

In a case-control study, persons with a given disease (the cases) and persons without the given disease (the controls) are selected; the proportions of cases and controls who have certain background characteristics or who have been exposed to possible risk factors are then determined and compared. Jennifer Kelsey (5)

A case-control study is an inquiry in which groups of individuals are selected in terms of whether they do (the cases) or do not (the controls) have the disease of which the etiology is to be studied, and the groups are then compared with respect to existing or past characteristics judged to be of possible relevance to the etiology of the disease. Brian McMahon and Thomas F. Pugh (6) persons who do not have that outcome or condition. The comparison is done for a number of determinants and potential exposures.

The basic approach of the case-control method is what the sociologists call ex-post facto or effect to cause "experiments." As Rothman and Greenland have stated, "The methodology of case-control studies has a sound theoretical basis, and as a means of increasing measurement efficiency in epidemiology, it is an attractive option" (7).

Using data on exposure frequencies in cases and controls, the case-control method is able to calculate a ratio of odds of exposure (OR) in cases and controls as a measure of association.

2.2.1 *Versatile, Informative, and Efficient Design*

Typically, a number of advantages and strengths have been ascribed to the case-control design. It is well suited to the study of rare diseases or those with long latency. It is relatively quick to mount and conduct and is reasonably inexpensive. The method requires comparatively few study subjects with very little risk to these subjects. In addition, the study allows us to test multiple hypotheses (evaluation of interaction and assessment of confounding factors) and assess exposures that are changing over time.

Thus, the method has both operational and conceptual strengths and advantages. On an operational level, these advantages include speed, cost, and the need for a limited number of study subjects.

On a conceptual level, and as a very versatile design, it is the method of choice to study diseases that are rare and have a long latency, and to test many hypotheses.

In summary, this is a design that is very informative (more cases and variables—information value) and very efficient (cost, time, rare disease).

2.3 CONTRADICTORY AND FALSE POSITIVE OUTCOMES

Since its first extensive uses in the 1950s, the case-control method has been the subject of much criticism but has withstood the test of time and has seen an exponential increase in its use.

The various weaknesses of the method that have been highlighted over the years include those that are common to all observational studies. All epidemiological studies have potential problems with inappropriate definitions of outcome or measurement of risk factors or study variables. A careful assessment of confounders is an integral part of any epidemiological study, whether experimental or case-based.

However, certain problems may be more common to case-control studies if appropriate provisions are not made to prevent them. One of the most difficult problems of the case-control method is the *selection of appropriate controls* that are picked from the same base population as the cases.

Considering that in many case-control studies we need to rely on the *recall* of the study subject to elicit past exposure information, the method may fail if actual recall does not reflect the past reality. Often past validation of information, even on a subgroup of the study subjects, may be close to impossible.

From a conceptual level, considering that we cannot calculate incidence rates for the various exposure groups in case-control studies, our inferences have to rely on the odds ratio (OR) as a measure of association and as an approximation of the relative risk.

Cumming and Kelsey have assessed the contradictory results obtained from case-control studies that tested the same relationship (8). Study quality was an issue for many, while others had more specific problems. These included failure to account for length of exposure, appropriate sample size, confounders, and period of latency. Some studies were selective in their presentation of study findings and had limited their citations to only a few other studies.

Swaen et al. compared 75 false positive studies to 150 true positive ones. The strongest factor that predicted a false positive study was the absence of a specific hypothesis. "Fishing expeditions" with no specific hypothesis had an OR of over 3 for showing false positive results (9).

2.4 INFERENCES FROM CASE-CONTROL STUDIES

As illustrated by the attached matrix (Box 2.1), at every step of our data collection process we have a sequence of inferential steps. For each of the different levels of data collection, these steps start with an assessment of potential biases in the methods and analyze the data for possible confounders and end with an evaluation of the significance and nature of the relationship.

A case-control study may have quite a few objectives and levels of concern. One needs to state at the outset the type of evidence expected to be achieved from the study. Most of the time, it is not difficult to make such a statement of expectation in the objectives of the study, if we assess the level of our knowledge regarding the problem at hand. An initial investigation of a health problem, with no major previously documented research and no specific hypotheses warrants an *exploratory*

Box 2.1 Epidemiologic methods and inferences matrix

| | *Inferences* | | |
Methods	Assess for bias	Review for confounders	Provide a causal model
Descriptive			
Mortality			
Morbidity			
Analytic			
Surveys			
Case-control			
Cohort			
Experimental			

approach with no expected finality of results regarding causality of associations. A study that follows up on a stronger set of evidence regarding a major hypothesis to be tested has an *analytic* purpose and will be scrutinized with a different set of criteria of evidence compared to exploratory studies.

A classic situation where our approach is usually exploratory is the study of a new condition that has not been studied previously or investigated as to a new spectrum of possible leads to etiology. Thus, the first case-control studies of Acquired Immunodeficiency Syndrome (AIDS) were able to identify some patterns of behavior that aided the transmission of the condition. Although these initial exploratory case-control studies did not provide the definitive evidence for the sexual transmission of the disease, they paved the way for more analytic investigations by delineating some directions to follow in gathering the evidence. In a case-control study on juvenile bone tumors from Austria, Frentzel-Beyme and colleagues interviewed 88 patients with bone tumors and their mothers as to a variety of risk factors, psychosocial factors, and factors occurring in early childhood and age 3, and gender-matched control groups. They reported a number of significant associations with childhood infections, breast feeding duration, and psychosocial factors. All of these associations could provide important leads for future investigations of the etiology of juvenile bone tumors (10).

Another situation where most investigations are exploratory is in conducting an outbreak investigation. In most such situations we have a number of hypotheses that can possibly explain transmission of the agent during the outbreak. An exploratory case-control study would test a number of these ideas and identify the more plausible ones. Similarly, exploratory analyses may be part of the case-control assessment of data from a disease surveillance system. This latter approach will be discussed further in the chapter on outbreak investigation.

Analytic or hypothesis testing can be done quite effectively using the case-control method. Whether a hypothesis is being tested for the first time or one is trying to replicate the findings of a previously investigated hypothesis, the case-control method is an efficient and effective method. The report on the observation in rats, that rubbing tobacco tar on the skin causes cancers of the urinary bladder in the animal, led Lilienfeld to test the hypothesis in humans (11). Based on available data from the epidemiological records of the Roswell Park Memorial Institute, he conducted a case-control study comparing cases of urinary bladder cancer with three different control groups. They were able to report the first human study on the subject and demonstrate a relationship between cigarette smoking and urinary bladder cancer within months of the animal studies.

In reviewing the inferential potential of a case-control study, we must first pay attention to the objectives that a particular study has set for itself. In many reports, it is not clearly stated what the inferential objectives of the study were at its beginning. As a result, confusion reigns as to contradictory findings, and the methodology of the case-control design is blamed as inappropriate for causal inferences. As Philip Cole stated in reviewing inferences in case-control studies, "the logical structure of the argument by which one deduces that an association is causal does not differ as a function of the source of the evidence" (12).

In examining the evidence from a case-control study, one needs also to consider disease classification issues. Disease classification is based on *etiological* or *manifestational* criteria. Asbestosis, tuberculosis, and posttraumatic stress disorder are conditions that are classified by etiology and the presence of—or exposure to—a necessary cause (i.e., asbestos, the tubercle bacillus, or major trauma) is a condition for the use of these diagnoses. Lung cancer, rheumatic fever, and schizophrenia are manifestational entities that are defined by the presence of certain clinical/pathological signs, symptoms, or other disease descriptors, which may evolve with time, as we better understand the condition. Thus, over time, a manifestational entity may evolve into an etiologic one as a major etiologic agent is identified. For example, the initial descriptive manifestational entity of AIDS evolved into an etiological entity following the discovery of the Human Immunodeficiency Virus (HIV) as the major etiological cause of the disease.

Diseases classified by etiology have one necessary cause that defines the condition. Thus, *Salmonella typhi* is accepted as *the* cause of typhoid fever and defines the illness. Manifestational conditions have no necessary cause. For example, smoking is the most important cause of lung cancer but one may develop lung cancer due to causes other than smoking. The diagnosis of lung cancer is conditional on clinical and pathological findings rather than by exposure to a particular etiological factor. Most etiological factors in epidemiology are not necessary. Hypercholesterolemia may be an important cause of coronary artery disease but the presence of high cholesterol is not necessary to classify a person as having coronary artery disease.

Thus, a case-control study of an etiologically defined entity is usually focusing on factors other than the defining etiology. In case-control studies of asbestosis or tuberculosis our primary concern is not to demonstrate the association between the disease and asbestos or the tubercle bacillus, but to assess the factors influencing exposure to these etiologies or the factors involved in the transmission of the disease agent. Hence, a case-control study of an etiologically defined condition may be as useful as a case-control study of a manifestational entity.

Cause is established in a continuing and evolving process. Every new study adds further evidence or negates existing evidence. Because of its efficiency, the case-control design is a method of choice to test a variety of hypotheses in this evolving process.

Concerns have been expressed as to the usefulness of data generated by this method for making inferences about causation because of design and data collection shortcomings in early case-control studies. Distrust has also been expressed in the method because it is backward looking, proceeding from effect to cause, while science in general proceeds from cause to effect. Sartwell and others have taken issue with this type of mistrust in the case-control design by highlighting the fact that important scientific theory has been developed using this effect to cause approach including the theory of the origin of species (13). Once we have conducted a case-control study that is methodologically valid and addresses potential shortcomings, data generated by this method should be as useful for making inferences as data from any other design. Philip Cole addressed this problem during a symposium by stating that "there is no fundamental flaw in the logical structure of the argument that allows us to assess causality from a case-control study" (14).

In reviewing evidence from case-control studies one can test it against the *criteria of judgment* that are frequently used in epidemiology. Except for time sequence, these criteria of judgment are not absolute, and should be used as guidelines in drawing conclusions about what are often complex relationships between presumed etiology and disease outcome.

The case-control design can address all the criteria of judgment. The method collects data across the *time span* of etiologic exposure ensuring that such exposure antedates outcome development within a reasonable period and is consistent with the latency of the condition. This is why every effort needs to be made to steer away from making the case-control study cross-sectional where it is not possible to decide on antecedence of presumed determinants to the occurrence of illness. The design of the study needs to assist us in separating the time of exposure from the onset of the disease or outcome.

The *strength* of the association, as assessed through our risk estimates is based on the analytic approaches we choose for the study. Reviewing *coherence* of the hypothesis with the known facts is related more with the initial hypothesis than the study design. If our study question makes theoretical, factual, and biological sense then coherence may be established to our satisfaction. Considering that most case-control studies deal with live persons, it is possible for these studies to incorporate tests for clinical as well as pathophysiologic mechanisms that try to explain the outcome.

In addition, because of its versatility of use under different conditions, the case-control method allows us to test for *specificity* of the association. Similarly, *consistency on replication* is easier to test in a case-control design than with other epidemiologic methods because of the built-in efficiencies of the method. If for example, a case-control study uses three different types of control groups from three different sources—such as a hospital control group, a neighborhood control group, and a sibling control group—and with each control group the study identifies the same level and direction of a relationship between disease and exposure, both the weight of our evidence for the association and the criterion of consistency upon replication are supported.

Judgment about causality is also influenced by our approach and philosophy regarding inferential reasoning. Inductive and deductive approaches to such reasoning are the two options that help us make judgments about causality. Epidemiological reasoning in its earlier expressions has been *primarily inductive*. According to Wade Hampton Frost "epidemiology is essentially an inductive science, concerned not merely with describing the distribution of disease, but equally or more with fitting it into a consistent philosophy" (15, p. 164). Thus, as an inductive process we develop hypotheses on the basis of a series of particular observations.

Sir Karl Popper and his followers in epidemiology have been the proponents of a more *deductive* approach to reasoning (16). For Popper, science advances by deduction alone and our reasoning on causality has to be based on a continuous process of trying to falsify the hypotheses that we put forth. Testability is the core function of this type of reasoning.

A hypothesis can never be proven. However, there are hypotheses that have never been rejected—so far.

The case-control design may be useful for inferential reasoning that uses both inductive and deductive approaches. In a case-control study what we observe are outcomes of some causal mechanism rather than the cause itself. We conceptualize about a hypothesis from multiple observations of people with and without the outcome. In an exploratory study where we are systematically reviewing various factors as potential etiologies for the outcome we may use primarily an inductive mode of reasoning whereby we synthesize data to generate a hypothesis.

Following the development of a hypothesis and at such a stage where a case-control study is more analytical and specific to testing a particular hypothesis, our approach may be deductive. We may try to study our data in a deductive mode not just through a process of falsification but also through one of assertion of findings that support our established hypothesis.

Judgment about causality and appropriate inferences needs to be made at three steps of a case-control or other epidemiological study: first, when developing a hypothesis, one can address most of these issues by ascertaining the existing store of knowledge and information regarding the presumed relationship(s); second, when designing the study, one may pay special attention to potential weaknesses in the strength of the argument for the hypothesis and make appropriate modifications in the design and in measurement of exposure; and third, when completing data analysis, one can address all the established criteria and provide a synthesis of judgment.

2.5 ANALYZING MORE COMPLEX ETIOLOGICAL MODELS

In assessing disease etiology, much of our effort is directed toward inferring the relationship of one etiological factor and an outcome. The reality is that in most situations the relationships between disease and etiology are more complex and may need to be addressed through more complex models. It is important to remember the "web of causation" that Brian MacMahon and colleagues described in their textbook (17). More than understanding the specific relationship of one factor and an outcome and trying to "isolate" that effect through multiple statistical manipulations—such as multivariate adjustments for confounders and an assessment of simple interactions—one needs to look at a disease process within complex systems of interacting forces. The current approach to multivariate etiologic analysis is, as described by Malcolm

Maclure, equivalent to identifying the specific etiological relationship within a subgroup that will explain the majority of the cases of the disease. Such a process of "purification" is currently done through stratification or multivariate analysis (18).

Past attempts to introduce methods of systems analysis to epidemiologic investigation include models from plant pathology: Kranz and Hau (19) proposed the use of the systems concepts in investigating epidemiologic problems. However, to date we have no actual examples of such systems analysis methods being applied to human epidemiology. As stated by Koopman and Lynch (20),

During much of the modern era of epidemiology, the analytic methods and causal models of epidemiology have been directed toward risk factor effects on individuals.... Analyses of how population level characteristics and patterns of exposure affect disease levels could be called "population system" epidemiology. In a system, in contrast to a "heap," the arrangement of elements makes a difference. When the pattern of exposures or connections between individuals in a population has the potential to make a difference to disease levels, we are dealing with a population system, not just a heap of individuals.

The case-control method has the capability to analyze etiologic relationships through multifaceted models and this is a major advantage of the method. It is possible to eliminate the effect of multiple confounders but also to test the interaction of a number of factors as we evolve toward understanding complex relationships. Strategies that one can use to study such complex models include

1. Developing a theoretical model that is able to synthesize our knowledge of the relationships involved, based on our current understanding of the disease in its ecological context.
2. Trying to validate and define individual relationships of etiological factors with the outcome as well as between these factors themselves.
3. Grouping factors and outcome(s) into subsets of interacting subsystems that make biological sense.
4. Developing coherent models for the interface of these subsystems. How do these models themselves interact with each other?
5. Testing the various assumptions made with these subsystems using the available data.
6. Revisiting the original comprehensive model of etiology and assessing its overall significance following empirical testing.

The case-control method can provide the database for each of these approaches outlined above. One can consider that the cases of disease belong to a system where things have gone wrong and our role as epidemiologists is to understand the processes that have made the system diseased by comparing a diseased subsystem with a system that is functioning normally.

Thus, one can study through the case-control method the structural characteristics of the system, such as socioeconomic and demographic characteristics, the health support system from family to health services, and nutritional and environmental characteristics. One can also study the actual processes that are of significance to the disease or to health. These may include various clinical tests of fitness of the system or subsystems.

Tactics used to study the role of multiple etiologies and disparate factors in such a systems approach include

1. Assessing the significance of each of the measured factors from a biological context.
2. Carrying out the usual multivariate analyses with a primary focus on studying the various presumed interactions between variables.
3. Evaluating whether risk for disease is increased with the development of new variables through scoring and other approaches.

2.6 INFERENCES AND PUBLIC POLICY

The case-control method should also be assessed as a tool that affects public policy. Influencing such policy is very dependent on the validity of the findings, the use of some standard methodologies to get the data or information, and the consistency of the observation with the known facts about the condition. The wealth of the information that the study provides will also be a critical factor in its assessment for public policy. For example, if our suspected etiological factor is not just presented as a stand-alone finding but as part of a complex model of etiological relationships and the mechanisms of action are already elucidated, it may have a better chance of being accepted and lead to more specific policy. If as a result of an interaction that we have identified, the effect is substantially limited to a subgroup of the population, then this may find better acceptance by policymakers and program developers because the intervention will be limited to the subgroup.

In considering issues of public policy, one needs to be concerned with generalizability. The case-control method allows us to study the problem from as representative a group as possible by targeting such groups of cases and controls from the population. As stated earlier, as a method it is easier to replicate without much effect or harm to the subjects involved.

As one considers issues of public policy, it is important to discuss the level of information that will have to be released to the public and particularly the conclusions to be made following an investigation. Often, investigators are prone to rush to the public news media prior to appropriate assessment of their study by the broader professional group or appropriate review of policy options. It is important to work with the old adage in mind: "Am I to do more harm than good?" In this case one needs to consider whether we are causing any harm by the release of the information.

As epidemiologists we need to strive toward obtaining the best database for our judgment. Data should be collected in a most objective fashion and its validity ascertained at every level. Although policy may influence interpretation, it should never influence the process of data collection and its analysis.

2.7 QUESTIONS FOR AN ASSESSMENT OF CASE-CONTROL STUDIES

The following questions are useful while designing a case-control study or evaluating one from the literature. They provide a road map that will be detailed in the chapters that follow and the reader may find it useful.

1. *Is there a clear definition of the problem under consideration?* Many studies lack such a clear definition. Is this study assessing factors influencing incidence or mortality?

2. *Is the definition of cases consistent with the definition of the problem?* A definition of cases needs to reflect the public health or medical problem the study is concerned with. Are we concerned with cerebrovascular accidents as a problem or the subset of hemorrhagic strokes? (See Chapter 3.)

3. *Are the controls selected from the same base population as the cases?* We need to have a clear idea of the base population from where we are selecting our cases (see Chapter 3).

4. *How valid is the measurement of the exposure(s) under consideration?*

5. *Is the process of selecting the cases and controls independent from the approach used to get information about exposure?* The lack of such independence between the two processes underlies the development of *biases* (see Chapter 3).

6. *Has the analysis considered the potential role of alternative explanations to the association under investigation?* One needs to consider whether the appropriate testing or handling was done for all potential *confounders* (see Chapters 6).

7. *Are there potential interactions between various factors that the authors have studied?* Interactions are other alternative explanations or hypotheses that we need to seek and identify if they exist (see Chapters 6).

8. *What is the information value of the published report with respect to the decision process in health services?* (See Chapters 1 and 2.)

REFERENCES

1. Diaz-Mitoma F, Vanast WJ, Tyrell DLJ. Increased frequency of Epstein-Barr virus excretion in patients with new persistent daily headaches. *Lancet.* 1987;1(8530):411-415.

2. Rose G. Sick individuals and sick populations. *Int J of Epidemiol.* 1985;14:32-38.

3. Sartwell PE. Retrospective studies: a review for the clinician. *Ann Intern Med.* 1974;81:381-386.

4. Cole P. Introduction. In: Breslow NE, Day NE (eds). *Statistical Methods in Cancer Research, Volume 1.The Analysis of Case-Control Studies.* Lyon: International Agency for Research on Cancer; 1980.14-40.

5. Kelsey JL, Thompson WD, Evans AS. *Methods in Observational Epidemiology.* New York: Oxford University Press; 1986:148-185.

6. McMahon B, Pugh TF. *Epidemiology: Principles and Methods.* New York: Little, Brown and Company; 1970.

7. Rothman KJ, Greenland S. *Modern Epidemiology.* Philadelphia: Lippincott-Rave; 1998.

8. Cumming RL, Kelsey JL. Case-control studies. *Int J Epidemiol.* 1989;18: 725-727.

9. Swaen GG, Teggeler O, van Amelsvoort LG. False positive outcomes and design characteristics in occupational cancer epidemiology studies. *Int J Epidemiol.* 2001;30:948-954.

10. Frentzel-Beyme R, Becher H, Salzer-Kuntschik M, Kotz R, Salzer M. Factors affecting the incident juvenile bone tumors in an Austrian case-control study. *Cancer Detection and Prevention.* 2004;28:159-169.

11. Lilienfeld AM. The relationship of bladder cancer to smoking. *Am J Public Health.* Nations Health 1964;54:1864-1875.

12. Cole P. The evolving case control study. *J Chronic Dis.* 1979;32(1-2):15-27.

13. Sartwell P. Comment. *J Chron Dis.* 1979;32:42-44.
14. Discussion following Drs. Cole and Acheson. *J Chron Dis.* 1979;32:30-34.
15. Frost WH. Epidemiology. Nelson Loose-Leaf System. *Public Health-Preventive Medicine*, Vol. 2, New York: Thomas Nelson & Sons; 1927. ch 7, 163-190.
16. Popper K. *The Logic of Scientific Discovery* (rev. ed.). New York: Harper & Row; 1968.
17. MacMahon B, Pugh TF, Ipsen J. *Epidemiologic Methods.* Boston: Little, Brown and Company; 1960.
18. Maclure M. Multivariate refutation of aetiological hypotheses in non-experimental epidemiology. *Int J Epidemiol.* 1990;19:782-787.

3

AVOIDING BIAS IN CASE AND CONTROL SELECTION

Haroutune K. Armenian

OUTLINE

This chapter aims to

1. provide a framework for understanding the development of bias in case-control studies;
2. define cases, given a health problem to be investigated;
3. identify sources of cases and controls to study a health problem;
4. assess the advantages and limitations of various types of controls within a specific study;
5. describe the strengths and limitations of matching as an approach to deal with confounding; and
6. identify various strategies to minimize or deal with selection bias.

3.1 AVOIDING BIAS

As information generated through epidemiologic studies needs to be valid and appropriate for making inferences about relationships between outcomes and their determinants, our design needs to minimize errors of measurement as well as control the effect of alternative explanations by confounders.

Little can be done about random errors except to ensure a large sample of the study population; however, we can avoid making systematic errors or biases at every step of the study. Thus, an important goal in designing a study—and in particular a case-control study—is to avoid biases. A number of design strategies also help us control the effect of confounders. In our epidemiologic investigation we try to get as close as possible to the truth and to get a true estimate of risk.

As presented in the previous chapter, the case-control method has characteristics that may lead to some difficulties and potential biases if we are not careful. Often we face a situation where sampling of the cases and controls needs to be done cross-sectionally. In a large number of other studies, data on cases and controls are collected separately, which may lead to biases being picked up through the different approaches. In addition, in a number of studies data on exposures is collected *retrospectively*, which may be responsible for a number of other biases of information.

In an analytic epidemiologic study, we seek to study the effect of some variable on a certain outcome. Two *independent* steps are essential for any such study: selecting the study population (cases and controls), and measuring exposure levels for these two study groups. Otherwise, the study may be rife with biased estimates of the exposure–outcome relationship.

Thus, in a case-control study, we may end up with such biased estimates of risk or association if *the process of selecting the cases and controls is not independent from the approach used to obtain exposure information*. Table 3.1 provides one approach of explaining bias by the principle of lack of independence of the two processes of selecting cases and controls and obtaining exposure information. If we are not able to achieve such independence then the validity of our results may be compromised (1). This principle of independence of the two processes

Table 3.1. The Effect of Independence of Selection of Cases and Controls from Exposure Assessment

If g, h, m, n represent the independent probabilities of selection on disease and exposure status such as

g = diseased, h = nondiseased, m = exposed, n = nonexposed

Then the four cells in our 2×2 table will be represented as:

	Cases	Controls
Exposed	gm A	hm B
Nonexposed	gn C	hn D

gm A represents the exposed cases
hm B represents the exposed controls
gn C represents the nonexposed cases
hn D represents the nonexposed controls

Thus, the estimated odds ratio(OR) in this 2×2 table will be represented by

$OR' = gmhn/gnhm \times OR = OR$

needs to be upheld at every step of the design and development of the case-control study.

As we consider the multiplicity of steps involved in the development and implementation of a case-control study, it is possible that some systematic error may bring about biased estimates of the association at any one of these steps. David Sackett has very well illustrated this point with his catalog of biases (2). In general, we deal with two major groups of biases: selection bias and information bias. Biases generated as a result of case and control selection or identification is *selection bias*, while those due to problems of exposure measurement or data collection processes are *information biases*. The result of these biases will lead to misclassification of case-control or exposure status.

3.2 CASE DEFINITION AND SELECTION

3.2.1 *Definition of the Problem and Cases*

The following two defining questions relate to the selection of cases:

1. Is there a clear definition of the problem under consideration?
2. Is the definition of the cases consistent with the definition of the problem?

Without a clear definition of the problem, it is not possible to visualize a clear case definition. Is the problem one of higher mortality or incidence? This relates to the *nature* of the problem. Is this a problem delineated in one geographic area or within one period of time? Is this problem limited to certain subgroups of the population? These questions relate to the *distribution* of the problem and help delimit the case definition based on the available information regarding such distribution. Thus, looking for answers to these questions will enhance our capability of making our study more targeted to its community of concern. For example, our definition of cases will be more focused if we target our problem as the incidence of myocardial infarction in young women over the past five years in Baltimore, rather than the more diffuse cardiovascular disease in Baltimore.

Once we have a specific definition of the problem under consideration, we need to ensure that our case definition is consistent with our problem definition. Our case definition, for the example above can be women with acute myocardial infarction from Baltimore aged less than 40 years. Thus, delineating our problem helps us to define our cases.

Decisions on case selection are determined by the problem under consideration but also by the specific hypothesis we want to test. If our hypothesis assumes that exposure to a new drug underlies new cases of the disease, then the cases we select need to come from a population where the drug is available. The *question* that governs the case-control investigation will, in a number of situations, determine our case definition. In an investigation of an epidemic of cholera where we are interested in identifying the mode of transmission of the infection *outside* the household, we would be wise to select as cases only the first cases in a household, since the other cases from the same household may be secondary to our primary case.

Another factor that affects case selection is the population we want to generalize to. Although our problem definition defines a frame within which cases are selected, certain problems may be quite complex and we may be limited to addressing the issue in a subset of the population to explain one facet of the problem only. For example, although we may need to study the relationship of radiation to lung cancer as a general population problem, our study may be circumscribed within an occupational group that has exposure to radiation. Thus, cases will be persons with lung cancer from that particular occupation and controls will be from the same occupation with no lung cancer.

The definition of a case needs to follow well-defined criteria. In addition to standard criteria that are established by specialized bodies, such as a definition by the American Rheumatism Association of a case of rheumatoid arthritis, we want to make sure that our definition is *unambiguous and reproducible*. The intent is to collect cases that are clinically similar to each other and that follow some agreed-upon definition, even if the sources for selecting them or the conditions under which we identify them are different. Using some standardized definition of the disease for cases also allows us to compare our results with other authors who have investigated the same problem previously.

The investigator needs to ascertain and document the evidence supporting the diagnosis in cases as well as any efforts made to rule out the presence of the disease in the control group. In reviewing data on diagnosis we need to assess whether cases and controls have undergone the appropriate laboratory or pathology tests for the disease under consideration. Some of the issues related to diagnostic ascertainment include

Are there any pathognomonic tests that serve to clinch the diagnosis? How many of the population have undergone this test? The presence of a positive result on a pathognomonic test makes a diagnosis, by definition, certain. An elevated level of thyroid stimulating hormone is pathognomonic for a diagnosis of hypothyroidism or, similarly, elevated fasting blood glucose is pathognomonic of diabetes. The absence of such a positive result in cases may make the case status possible or probable depending on the other evidence for the disease in the selected person.

Should there be a review of the slides or the tests that were conducted to establish the diagnosis? As part of a diagnostic validation effort for their case-control study of endometrial cancer and estrogen use, Antunes et al. confirmed the histologic report or the operative report in a subsample of 55 of their cases of endometrial cancer from Baltimore (3).

How do we handle the situation where there are certain missing elements from the diagnostic evidence for some of the patients? In many studies this situation is handled primarily at the level of data analysis, by testing the hypothesis separately in the two groups with different levels of diagnostic certainty. One can compare the results of the analysis of the subset of cases with incomplete diagnostic validation with those that have a full diagnostic ascertainment. If the results are similar in both groups then there is less of a chance for misclassification due to case-control status.

For multiple sources of pathology information and multiple methods used to establish the diagnosis in the cases, what is the level of variability between different tests and the agreement/disagreement between multiple observers and methods of diagnosis?

Case selection will determine decisions on control selection. Thus, as a first step in the conduct of a case-control study, case definition and selection will affect all the other steps that follow.

3.2.2 Sources of Cases

Table 3.2 lists a number of sources where cases may be identified. These include existing sources of medical care, various information systems and registries, and other institutions or facilities where people with illness are identified and recorded. Cases may be identified through special surveys and screening programs conducted in the community or population-based registries. The sources of cases can affect our ability to generalize to the population at risk. If our sources cover all potential cases in the reference population, then this may assist in the computation and derivation of rates that relate to the whole population. In considering most of these sources of cases, we need to remember that they are usually developed for administrative and program management purposes and may have serious shortcomings when used for rigorous research.

Table 3.2. Sources of Cases

1. People seeking care
   - Patients at specific medical care facilities
   - Hospital discharges
   - Clinics

2. From community and other registries
   - Specialized registries
   - Other information systems

3. Other sources
   - Schools
   - Military
   - Prepaid Health Plans
   - Community Surveillance
   - Cases in a cohort—nested

3.2.3 Issues Related to Case Selection

3.2.3.1 *Misclassification of cases.* For most diseases we deal with a spectrum of severity of the condition. At one end of the spectrum we have normal persons and at the other end we have people with the incapacitating or fatal forms of the condition. While identifying cases, it is very important to define the stage at which cases are selected since the severity of the condition may affect our assessment of the association between exposure and outcome. Fried and Pearson (4) evaluated a sample of patients undergoing arteriography to assess whether associations between exposure or risk factors and disease are affected by changes in the arteriographic definition of absence of disease. Their analysis showed that the prevalence of disease risk factors was higher with increasing atherosclerosis. They concluded that including subclinical or moderate atherosclerosis might weaken the estimates of associations of disease and risk factors. Since most diseases have a large subclinical component, we may also need to look for potentially misclassified cases in the controls. Such a problem will not be very serious if the disease under consideration is rare and thus we are dealing with a few misclassified controls. However, in a condition like benign prostatic hyperplasia (BPH), where over a third of men over the age 70 may have the condition, controls selected from the population for the cases of BPH may have major misclassification issues if the subclinical condition of benign prostatic hyperplasia is not excluded through some examination of the selected controls.

3.2.3.2 *Prevalent cases.* For a case-control study, selection of incident cases is preferred to selection of prevalent cases. Prevalence includes information on survival and remission; prevalent cases are those who have survived the condition up to that point in time. If survival is in some way related to whether the person is exposed to the factor under consideration, then the two processes of case selection and exposure may not be independent and we may end up with some biased estimates of the association. Prevalence is equal to incidence times duration. A ratio of two incidence rates (relative risk = a ratio of the incidence in exposed to the incidence in the nonexposed) is equivalent to a ratio of two prevalence rates if the duration of the disease does not differ between those who are exposed and those nonexposed. For example, if exposure to cigarettes improves survival following the development of lung cancer, then by using the prevalent cases we may overestimate the level of the association between cigarette smoking and lung cancer because of the survival advantage due to the exposure. Similarly, if exposure to cigarettes shortens survival following the development of lung cancer, then by using the prevalent cases we may underestimate the level of the association between cigarette smoking and lung cancer because of the survival disadvantage due to exposure.

Thus, in a case-control study one can use prevalent cases if the duration of the disease is not affected by exposure status. Then again, there may be practical considerations for not using prevalent cases in case-control studies. These include

1. difficulty in delineating antecedence of exposure in prevalent cases. In a chronic, longstanding illness it may be difficult to define the time relationship between the exposure and the onset of the illness.
2. a lack of recency or freshness in the history of events and exposures when comparing prevalent cases to incident cases.

One advantage of prevalent cases is their availability; they may require much less effort when searching in multiple sources and for diagnostic assessment than incident cases. It is also important to consider situations where all cases are prevalent, such as all conditions present at birth or those detected as an ancillary finding during a diagnostic or screening examination. Enuresis is a condition present at birth whereby every individual is enuretic at birth; in a case-control study we might be concerned with continuing enuresis after a certain age and what factors help maintain the condition. Thus, our study is not any more a study of factors leading to the incidence of enuresis but a study of factors that help maintain enuresis in its prevalent form. Congenital malformations are another set of conditions where almost all cases are prevalent since they exist at birth.

For many diseases the bulk of the cases are identified through a diagnostic or screening examination. Examples of such conditions include asymptomatic uterine fibroids discovered during laparoscopy, or abdominal aneurysms discovered through routine X-rays or other procedures.

As with any other potential source of error, it is worthwhile to assess the size of the effect or impact a prevalence-incidence bias may have on the study results in any study that uses prevalent cases.

3.2.3.3 Dating the onset of the illness for cases, which becomes an important consideration in view of the potential for prevalence-incidence bias. Usually, we date the onset of the disease in the cases from the date a diagnosis is established. However, in chronic diseases, symptoms may be present months and sometimes years prior to an established diagnosis. In other conditions the actual onset may be very difficult to determine. Our predominant concern is to make sure that the identified exposures preceded the earliest symptoms.

3.2.3.4 Changes in case definition and ascertainment over time. Definitions and ascertainment technology evolve over time. The changes that may affect such definitions include

1. A new system of international classification of diseases and causes of death or a redefinition of the condition by a professional or governmental group. Prior to data collection, it will be important to review the cases regarding how these redefinitions would affect identifying and classifying our cases.
2. Newer technologies may make it possible for the cases to be discovered at a much earlier stage than usual, and access to these newer technologies may differ across time periods and across facilities for members within the group of cases. If stage and severity are affected by exposure, we may get a different assessment of risk depending on the period of time or the sources of identification of cases.

3.2.3.5 Exposure and case definition. In defining our cases one needs to consider whether exposure should play any role in such definitions. This is one of the most serious issues of case selection, and situations where such considerations of etiology are necessary include

1. When cases of a disease defined by etiology, such as tuberculosis, need to be exposed to the defining etiological factor, such as tubercle bacillus. Case-control investigations in such etiologically

defined conditions will focus not on identifying the primary causal factor but aim at studying its method of transmission in a particular context.

2. When cases are needed to investigate a subtype of exposure or a subgroup of exposure to provide some understanding of mechanisms of linkage between broader exposure and disease. If John Snow had to pursue further his work on the transmission of cholera by trying to demonstrate whether a subsource of the water was the main culprit for the epidemic of cholera or to test whether some important contributing factors exist that help in such transmission, he could conduct a case-control study limited to users of the polluted water of Southwark and Vauxhall companies. Once he had established that the polluted water provided by these companies caused the cholera, Snow's next step could have been to question why not everyone drinking the polluted water developed the disease. Selecting both cases and controls from a subgroup of exposure, that is the population using the polluted water, could establish that water from a particular stream (s) or pump (s) is placing people at higher risk. One needs to note that this type of use of exposure information for case and control definition is symmetrical in that both cases and controls are assumed to be exposed to the polluted water.

3. When cases are selected to study etiological factors that are very strongly related to disease, as with cigarette smoking. Where smoking is an exposure that may overwhelm the elucidation of other risk factors, we may like to limit the selection of both our cases and controls from nonsmokers. This may allow us to detect some of the other factors that are related to the disease.

These are a few situations where information about etiology may affect our case definition. A controversy developed in the 1980s as to whether the cases and controls need to be collected on the basis of opportunity for exposure. As we develop eligibility criteria, we hope to identify both cases and controls that have an opportunity for exposure. If we include too many persons who have no opportunity for exposure, then we are diluting the effect of an association and biasing our estimates of the odds ratio toward one. As a simple example, in a study of oral contraceptive use and peripheral vascular disease, cases and controls need to be selected from a period of time when oral contraceptives became available in the study community to make the study meaningful and for efficient use of resources. Here again, we may be dealing with a situation where biased results may be obtained if the process of case and control selection is not independent of the process of getting exposure information.

3.2.3.6 *Exclusion and inclusion criteria.* As in the last example it is important that if we decide on incorporating some inclusion or exclusion characteristics within our case definition, such as limiting the cases to a certain subgroup of nonsmokers, identical exclusion or inclusion criteria must be applied to our definition of the controls.

3.2.3.7 *Case subgroup analysis.* When subgroups have well-established clinical or pathological characteristics—and if we are dealing with a large enough sample size—it is worthwhile to conduct analyses of these subgroups as separate case groups and compare them with their controls, as well as with the results obtained from the broader case group and the other subgroups of the disease. This will answer the question as to whether these subgroups have an epidemiologically different set of determinants. For example, in a case-control study of stroke, it is important to separate the group into hemorrhagic versus thrombotic disease. Hiller et al. (5) studied the subgroups of cataracts as to their epidemiological characteristics and reported that "cortical cataracts were more common in women and more often found in locations with increased UV-B radiation counts than either nuclear or posterior subcapsular cataracts." In a case-control study of 558 histologically confirmed epithelial ovarian cancer cases and 607 population controls, Tung et al. (6) have demonstrated that there were significant differences between the various histological types of epithelial ovarian cancers. They concluded that the various histological types of ovarian cancer were etiologically distinct.

3.2.3.8 *Limited availability of cases.* In situations where the disease is very rare, a number of approaches can be used to make a case-control study feasible. In such situations, we may reconsider the stringency of the diagnostic criteria or we may think about incorporating in the study cases from broader time periods, a variety of sources, and locations.

3.2.3.9 *Diagnostic bias.* Underlying such bias is the suspicion that our ascertainment of the disease is influenced by our knowledge of exposure. If a person is given estrogens, then that person receiving estrogens may be under closer diagnostic scrutiny and surveillance than someone who is not given estrogens. As a result of such bias, the estimated odds ratio may be spuriously elevated because more cases are identified because of their exposure rather than independently through the natural history of the illness.

3.2.3.10 *Summary.* In summary, the following are some guidelines for case selection:

- Remember that problem definition determines case definition
- Consider alternative sources and approaches for case selection
- Validate the diagnosis of cases according to accepted criteria
- Analyze data for various levels of certainty of diagnosis
- Assess the impact of prevalent cases in the study population
- Assess the role, if any, of exposure in the definition or selection of cases and controls.

3.3 CONTROL SELECTION

3.3.1 Overview

Decisions on the selection and identification of the control group are probably some of the most critical in the conduct of a case-control study. The control group provides a reference or comparison group to the cases: it does not just represent a group of people who are not diseased or who do not have the outcome of interest, but rather it is a group that shares with the cases a potential for exposure in the past and for much of the time period under consideration. In a clinical research environment, one would compare people with the disease with "normal" controls that as a group will provide a measure of the baseline expected physiological values or processes. The problems with defining normality have been discussed in detail by Edmond Murphy in a series of articles (7,8). Thus, if we are measuring some hormonal changes in patients with hypertension, we will compare the values of these hormones in these patients with those same values in some healthy volunteers, usually younger persons. Such a comparison may be fraught with problems because it does consider the potential selection biases and the role of confounders. In an epidemiological case-control study the selection of controls needs to be scrutinized with some of these potential problems in mind.

The major concern for control selection is that the controls need to be selected from the *same base population* as the cases. If the controls are to provide an estimate of the exposure in the population in the absence of the outcome or disease, then they need to come from the same base population where our inferences about the cases are going to be made. Controls represent the population at risk for the development of the disease or outcome. Schlesselman states that "the control series is intended to provide an estimate of the exposure rate that would be expected to occur in the cases if there was no association between the study disease and exposure" (9).

If the controls are to be used as a comparison group to make inferences about the relationship between outcomes and exposure, then *comparability* of the controls to cases becomes another important dimension to consider in our selection process.

Thus, in selecting our controls in a case-control study, we need to address both of these concerns of comparability and generalizability. A high level of comparability assures the validity of the findings and a valid study can be carried out in a highly restricted group of individuals.

3.3.2 Operational Factors

Over the years, and at a more applied level of the case-control method, efforts have been made to develop standard approaches to the selection of controls in certain investigative situations. For example, in a case-control investigation of an outbreak, one may develop a standard approach for selecting neighborhood controls for a certain category of food and waterborne diseases. Although such standardization may assist methodologically unsophisticated epidemiological personnel with using the case-control method, as well as allow comparability of investigations across many outbreaks, unique and peculiar aspects in any investigation may require making special decisions to elucidate the relationships under consideration. We discuss below some of the operational factors that affect control selection.

3.3.2.1 *Sources of cases.* Using the same data sources to identify both cases and controls improves our confidence that both cases and controls are coming from the same base population. If all cases are identified from pathology records, then using pathology records to select controls from other patients who had a pathology exam but turned out not to have the case condition assures that the same selection patterns have been applied for both case and control identification.

3.3.2.2 *Availability of a sampling frame or roster.* At times it may be difficult to define a sampling frame from which one can select at random a group of controls. In the absence of such a roster, one may embark on developing one or using a matching process in the selection of controls.

3.3.2.3 *Availability of controls.* When the cases are at such an extreme of a distribution, it may not be possible to find adequate numbers of controls to select from in the nondiseased group. For example, if our cases are all in their eighth or ninth decade of life, we may not have much choice for identifying nondiseased or nonaffected controls in those age groups.

3.3.2.4 *Cost efficiency and accessibility.* Cost of identifying and collecting data from controls as well as access to potential controls may create serious problems in our decision process.

3.3.2.5 *Timing of control selection.* Controls may be selected from all other noncases at the point in time when the case develops the disease. Another approach allows for selecting controls after all cases have been identified in the population under consideration during the study period. The first of these selection processes is called *incidence-density* selection of the controls while the second is called *cumulative-incidence* method of selecting controls. It is preferable to select controls as the cases are occurring; however, in nested and retrospective case-control studies, all the cases may have already been identified in the population and there is no point in trying to select controls using the incidence-density sampling. The advantages and potential problems with these two selection processes will be discussed later.

3.3.2.6 *Controls with diseases associated with the exposure.* The accepted practice is to exclude such controls that are associated with the exposure. For example, should we exclude patients with lung cancer as controls from a study of chronic bronchitis and cigarette smoking? Such misclassification may be more important for controls selected from a single disease group than from controls selected from multiple disease conditions where one type of bias does not affect the results significantly in all study groups. This is one of the more difficult problems of hospital-based case-control studies. How large an association will produce a bias that will affect the significance of the association? This question needs to be addressed individually for each study under such circumstances.

3.3.2.7 *Controls for dead cases.* As controls for such cases have a high probability of being alive, data collected for the cases will come from a different source than for controls. Information on case exposure will rely very heavily on proxy respondents, while the controls who are alive may be interviewed personally. The options in such a situation include interviewing a proxy for controls for each dead case, or conducting dual interviews of the study subject and the proxy for all controls. Our concern would be with any resulting biases. If dying is associated with exposure, then our estimate of the odds ratio may be biased. Howe (10) emphasizes that the use of dead controls for dead cases will allow comparability of data quality between the comparison groups, particularly with regard to data on confounders. In his example of a study of radom exposure and lung cancer within a cohort in Howe's study, the cases were 89 miners who had died of lung cancer. The cohort lacked data on cigarette smoking as a major confounder. Howe traced proxy respondents for these cases as well as for their 213 selected controls who had died of causes other than lung cancer. A nested case-control study was conducted with these study groups of dead cases and dead controls to assess the role of smoking as a confounder in this relationship using similar approaches for tracing and data collection through proxy interviewing for both study groups. Falbo et al. (11) conducted a case-control study of homicides in children and adolescents in Recife, Brazil, by comparing 255 homicide victims under 20 years of age and 255 neighborhood controls matched by age and gender. For both cases and controls, interviews were conducted through a questionnaire with the closest relative.

3.3.3 Matching

The primary reason for matching is to establish case-control comparability as to confounders. For the few variables that we match on, we hope to achieve similarity of distribution between cases and controls. Based on the model of experimental controlled trials, the idea of matching cases and controls is very attractive since it forces comparability between the study groups. However, matching is not an efficient approach for establishing comparability since we can match on very few confounders at a time, such as age and gender. Alternatively, in a multivariate analysis, we may be able to adjust for a larger number of confounders and in clinical trials comparability is established on all the known as well as the unknown confounders through randomization.

3.3.3.1 *Matching decisions.* Matching cases and controls on some characteristic may involve more than our variable of interest. Thus, matching on occupation establishes comparability not just on a certain set of environmental exposures associated with occupation but also on socioeconomic status, and on such lifestyle patterns as exercise and smoking. Every time we match on a variable, we need to assess that we are not matching on the exposure of interest. However, in some situations we may be interested in establishing comparability for certain variables that present difficulties in measuring or obtaining data. Information on occupation may be readily available and we may use the data as a proxy measure for lifestyle or socioeconomic status if we have difficulty in getting data on the latter variables. Thus, matching on a factor as a proxy variable can also be used to establish comparability on another variable. For example, we may use matching on education as a proxy for socioeconomic factors or nutritional status.

An advantage of matching is the improvement in the precision of our estimate of the measure of association. In some situations, and with a confounder with a strong effect on the association of interest, it is possible to obtain two different extremes of distribution by confounder between the cases and the controls. Thus, our measure of association will reflect the skewed distributions of the confounders rather than the exposure factor. Matching by the confounder will help us identify a more precise effect of our variable of interest. By forcing comparability of the two groups with regard to the confounder we have minimized its effect.

Another reason for using matching is to select controls from the same population group as cases. For example, if we match on residence or workplace, we may be able to align controls to the same subgroup of interest as the cases, even if these factors are not confounders.

Decisions on matching and control selection need to involve the following:

Ascertaining that the matched variable is a confounder by studying the relationship of the variable with the outcome (case-control status) as well as the exposure under study and that the presumed confounder is not on the pathway between the exposure and the outcome at an intermediate phase. It is not justifiable to match for a variable that is related only to exposure or outcome. Also, if we are able to measure the confounder, then we may not need to match since we are able to address the confounder in the analysis by adjustment. Matching may be limited to variables possible to measure.

Deciding the number of controls to match to the cases. Up to four to five controls per case increases the power of the test. In a study with a large number of cases we may not even need a full complement of controls. The advantage of more than one control group will be discussed later in this chapter.

Establishing the number of variables on which to match depends on practical considerations as well as the extent to which we care to establish close comparability. It becomes very cumbersome to match on more than a few variables at a time. Also, the more we make the case and control groups comparable the less opportunity we will have to observe differences on some of the variables of interest.

3.3.3.2 *Potential problems associated with matching decisions* are given below:

Inability to estimate the effect of the matched variable on the outcome. If we match on gender then we are making the case and control groups similar as to the proportion of males and females. Thus, we eliminate our ability to observe differences in gender between the two study groups.

Potential cost increase. Individual matching may increase the complexity of study management as well as cost. If we decide to match on gender and 5-year age groups, then we need to search through a roster of potential controls within these limits of gender and age for every case we identify. This is one reason that *group matching* is preferable to individual matching. The effort needed to identify persons to match, and sometimes the limited availability of such persons, may substantially reduce the number of available controls for our study with resulting loss of power in our ability to detect an association.

Loss of precision. Although one reason for matching is to increase the precision of the study, there may be actual loss of precision in the study if matching is done inappropriately on a variable that is not a direct or indirect confounder.

Manipulating the distribution of exposure for the controls. Controls should not be matched on the cases to the extent that they are forced to have a different distribution of exposure than they would under normal circumstances. Matching may manipulate our exposure assessment indirectly so that the control group does not reflect exposure in the population in the absence of disease. Over the years, for example, a concern has been expressed that if we carry matching too far (i.e., matching on variables that may not be confounders), we may lose precision because of an increased number of concordant matched pairs. In addition, at times we may end up making cases and controls similar with respect to the distribution of the exposure of interest. This phenomenon has been described as *overmatching*. One example of overmatching occurs when we match the controls to the cases on an antecedent of the disease. Matching cases and controls on specific categories of occupation in a study of radiation and lung cancer may force a similarity of exposures to radiation between cases and controls. It is also possible that if we match on too many variables we match indirectly on the exposure of interest. If we match the cases and controls on age, gender, occupation, education, and alcohol use simultaneously, we may indirectly match on smoking if the latter is our exposure of interest. Since in a matched analysis we are interested in the discordant pairs of cases and controls, extremes of matching, such as described here, may result in more concordant than discordant pairs, thus moving our estimate of the odds ratio toward one.

Matching on categories of the confounder that are too broad. If matching is done on categories of the confounder that are too broad, we may be unsuccessful in eliminating the effect of the confounding variable since the resultant distribution of cases and controls within these broad categories may allow the effect of the confounder to continue. This is the potential risk of *residual confounding* that may need to be addressed at both the design and analysis phases. De Vries et al. re-examined the data from two case-control studies on the association between the use of statins and the risk of fractures and obtained different results in the same data base. This difference of the results between the two studies was reduced when matching of cases and controls in one of the studies was done by year of birth, rather than by 5-year age band. They explained the discrepancies of results between the two studies by residual confounding by a matching variable and different definitions of the exposure window (12).

Not maintaining matching during analysis. When cases are matched to controls, pairing as established initially needs to be maintained throughout the analysis of the study. Ignoring matching in the analysis may move our odds ratio estimates toward one.

Matching can be done at two levels: individual or group. In individual matching we aim to establish comparability at the individual level to obtain such comparability at the group level. The result of effectively matching a case on age and gender to one or more controls is to make the case and control groups similar with regard to age and gender. However, if we aim to establish comparability between a case and a control on more than two variables, it may become problematic to identify a control with three similar variables to the case unless we have an unlimited pool to choose from. We have to consider that comparability could be effectively established through multivariate adjustment.

For group, frequency, or category matching, cases and controls are matched within broad characteristics as a group and the matching effort is focused on establishing group comparability between the cases and controls rather than establishing similarity between individual cases and controls. In this approach one needs information on the distribution of cases with regard to the confounders. Controls are selected according to the distribution of the cases and the result should be a distribution of the confounding variable that is proportionally the same as the distribution of the cases for that same variable. As stated earlier, group matching should result in fewer problems with loss of data and sample size than individual matching.

3.3.4 Issues of Control Selection

3.3.4.1 *Numbers and type of controls.* In general, we do not need to select more than one control group unless there are possible shortcomings with the controls we are selecting. For example, if we suspect that our hospital-based controls may increase the likelihood of a selection bias, then we may decide to select a second group of controls from the community, such as neighborhood controls, that are not subject to the selection biases of the hospital-based group. With a second group of controls we may enhance the strength of our argument with our findings if our analysis yields the same results for the two different control groups. However, in case of a discrepancy between the two control groups as to the findings in the study, the reason for the discrepancy between the two control groups may shed light on the processes underlying the development of the disease. Multiple groups of controls serve both as an approach to check on biases and to assess the consistency of the association. Sulheim et al. studied the protective effect of helmet use for head injuries in alpine skiers and snowboarders in a case-control study at eight major Norwegian alpine resorts (13). They compared their 578 cases of head injuries to two groups of controls: noninjured controls interviewed at the bottom of the main ski lift at each resort during peak hours and injured controls with injuries other than the head. Wearing a helmet was associated with a 60% reduction in the risk of head injury and the results were similar for analyses with all control groups. Linet and Brookmeyer (14) reviewed 106 case-control studies of cancer and identified 9 that used more than one control group. According to the authors, "reasons for using more than one control group varied, but generally included one of the following: to permit comparisons with other studies that used hospital controls, to address potential inadequacies of the other control group of the study, or to evaluate potential bias (selection, detection, or use of a particular source of information about exposure)."

3.3.4.2 *Misclassification.* Misclassification of early or undetected case disease in controls needs to be addressed for a number of conditions. In conditions that have a large pool of undetected disease, it will be important to assess the potential for misclassification. Thus, it is always preferable to have the controls undergo some similar level of diagnostic assessment as the cases of the disease to rule out undetected pathology. In a few case-control studies, both cases and controls are selected from the same group of persons undergoing a diagnostic test. For example, in a case-control study of abdominal aortic aneurysms, Blanchard et al. (15) selected their cases and controls from people undergoing abdominal radiologic procedures. Cases were those showing an aneurysm, while controls had undergone the same procedures as the cases for a number of suspected other conditions.

3.3.4.3 *Identifying more specific etiologies.* We are often interested in identifying etiologies that go beyond some broad observation of an association. In such situations we may use a case-control study where both cases and controls are exposed to the broader etiological factor. The specific question that one tries to address in such studies relates to identifying some factors that can explain why a number of persons who are exposed do not develop the disease. For example, it is a known fact that people who are homozygous for familial hypercholesterolemia are at a high risk to die young from coronary artery disease. A case-control study was performed comparing cases of coronary artery disease (CAD) and controls without clinical CAD whereby both cases and controls had familial hypercholesterolemia. The two groups differed significantly as to the presence of tendon xanthomas as well as an arcus senilis in the eye (16). In another study, Thompson et al. (17) tested the effectiveness of bicycle safety helmets in preventing head injuries in the Seattle, Washington area. Both their cases and controls were bicyclists. Although the cases had head injuries, the controls were identified from the same emergency rooms as the cases, but from bicyclists who had problems other than head injuries that led them to the emergency room.

3.3.4.4 *Developing a pool of controls for multiple studies.* In large research programs where multiple case-control studies may be conducted, one may develop such a pool of available controls, although a number of problems can exist with such a pool. These include nonconcurrent interviewing of cases and controls, and controls that may not have all the required information for the particular study of interest.

3.3.5 *Types and Sources of Controls*

Two major strategies in designing a case-control study affect the selection of controls and analysis of the investigation. Case-control studies using an *incidence-density* approach of sampling select controls from all eligible noncases at the point of incidence of cases. Thus, when a case of disease occurs, controls are selected from the rest of the population of all eligible controls at that point in time. This method of selection of controls would allow some controls that have no disease to develop it on follow-up. The advantage for such an incidence-density selection strategy of controls is that it establishes comparability between cases and controls as to follow-up time for the detection of disease. Thus, this approach will allow the investigator to estimate relative rates of the disease as it relates to exposure. However, for a disease that is not very rare, there may be some misclassification of cases as controls. Some of the controls may turn up as cases on follow-up. In a follow-up of controls participating in case-control studies, Koch et al. (18) reported that over a period of five years, 4% of the controls had developed the case diseases of prostate cancer and melanoma.

In *cumulative-incidence* case-control studies, the approach to sampling of controls is to select all the cases and the controls at the end of a well-defined period of study. Cases identified during that period are selected, as well as controls that have not developed the disease or condition at the end of that period. Thus, controls are no more at risk for the disease during the study period. The odds ratio calculated from such a study is an approximation of relative risk. In practical terms, there is little effect between these two strategies regarding our ability to make inferences in case-control studies if the disease is rare. In settings where the disease is rare, our estimates of odds ratio, relative rate, and risk ratio will be similar for both *incidence-density* and *cumulative-incidence* sampling approaches.

The following section presents the uses and some of the problems of various types of controls.

3.3.5.1 *General population.* Controls selected from the general population have a major advantage of being representative of the broader community. Thus, the results of the study with such controls should be more generalizable and can make some of the strongest arguments in support of the study findings. Also, data generated from population-based controls may provide us a truer picture of the frequency of exposure in the community, which may be very useful for our estimates of attributable risk. An example of controls from the general population is the neighborhood controls—starting from the address of a case, one identifies through a random process a neighbor without the disease and with the desired characteristics for the control group. It is useful to note that such controls are indirectly matched to the cases on many characteristics identified in that neighborhood. When selecting such controls, it is good practice to get data on length of residence within the neighborhood for both cases and controls, since length of residence may act as a confounding variable. Some potential problems with such population controls include the possible lack of cooperation among the individuals selected as controls in their residences, compared to those identified through the health-care system; and the possible expense of identifying and interviewing such controls. Probably the best approach for selecting population controls occurs when we have access to a roster of the base population and we are able to randomly select a sample of controls from that roster. In the absence of a roster one may use maps of the community under investigation and randomly sample households and buildings to potentially identify a control of interest to the study.

3.3.5.2 *Hospital patients.* Controls from other patients admitted to the hospital from which the cases are selected have the advantages of accessibility, a similar frame of mind to the cases as a result of hospitalization, and having undergone selection processes similar to the cases. However, there may be few difficulties with such controls, including obtaining consent of the treating physician prior to approaching the patient. Hospitalized patients are not typical of the general population. We may have difficulties in our inferences if we want to project our study to a broader group than those hospitalized. On a conceptual level, case control-studies with hospital patient controls may be fraught with selection biases due to a variety of issues related to differential access and admission to the hospital for various subgroups of the population or for various diagnostic subcategories. Selection of controls from the same hospital as the cases may also be on the exposures that are under investigation. Selecting controls from the hospital will bias our comparison groups toward the more exposed in the population if the control diseases are related to the exposure. For example, if the exposure under consideration is smoking or alcohol, then there is a high probability that many of the controls admitted for other diseases have conditions that are associated with smoking and alcohol. Moritz et al. (19) tested whether selecting hospital controls versus population controls "would influence conclusions regarding risk factors for hip fractures." Cases were 425 persons with hip fracture. Two different groups of controls were tested: 312 hospital controls and 454 community controls. Community controls were similar to community-dwelling elderly women, whereas hospital controls were sicker and more likely to be current smokers. The authors concluded that community controls comprised the more appropriate control group in case-control studies of hip fracture in the elderly (19).

3.3.5.3 *Random digit dialing* (RDD). This can be used to screen and identify potential controls and to interview them in person, or both to identify and interview controls over the telephone using the RDD system. If the interview is conducted over the telephone, a household visit can be avoided. However, this method of interviewing is restricted to those with a telephone, and those with multiple telephones may have a higher probability of being selected and interviewed. The major advantage of such controls is the random approach that is used to select a group from the broader community. With the current restrictions established on access to persons who are available for interviewing by the use of answering machines and other controls of communication methods, this approach has become more difficult for selecting controls and interviewing the study population. The method involves obtaining a list of all telephone area codes and prefixes in the study area, getting the telephone numbers of cases, and generating a list of random numbers that has the same area code and prefix as the case and have the last few digit numbers selected at random. These telephone numbers are used to identify controls that are coming from the same study area as the cases. Within the same study and in the same community Olson et al. (20) compared controls recruited from RDD and controls recruited at random from a commercial database of a mailing list. Both control groups were similar to each other in terms of sociodemographic characteristics and also on some of the study variables of oral contraceptives, nulliparity, and religion. The control groups differed significantly from the cases on the latter three variables. However, the commercial database was able to identify only 28% of the cases, raising the question of whether controls selected through this database came from the same base population as the cases. The authors concluded that the use of a commercial database provided a control group similar to the cases as to sociodemographic distribution at a considerable cost saving compared to the controls recruited through RDD. In another study, Olson et al. (21), compared interviews from a sample of the population of Oswego County, NY, identified through RDD as potential controls, with the data from a private census of 15,563 men and women aged 40 to 74 from the same county. For most variables there were no differences in the distribution between the two comparison groups including all sociodemographic variables. However, the RDD group had a slightly higher proportion of people who had various screening tests. The authors cautioned users of RDD-identified control groups of the possibility of selection-detection biases when using such controls.

3.3.5.4 *Spouse, sibling, friend, classmate, coworker.* Each of these controls establishes similarity with the cases on one or more characteristic. Thus, a spouse control is similar to the case with regard to household characteristics, nutrition, lifestyle, and familial exposures, while a sibling control is similar to the case as to genetics and early life experiences. A friend is similar to the case as to demographic characteristics and lifestyle, while a classmate or coworker is similar to the case with respect to education and other socioeconomic factors. These controls are useful as an additional control group to test particular hypotheses and they are also relatively easy to identify as controls. However, these controls need to be named by the cases and often a case may be reluctant to name a friend or colleague for such a role because of some potential inconvenience to the person. In a case-control study investigating a genetically determined metabolic characteristic, Shaw et al. (22) reported that only 11 of 23 cases named at least one friend as a potential control. Spouses and siblings are usually available as controls, while for friend, classmate, or coworker controls one may ask the case to name a number of their friends or coworkers. The investigator can then select at random one of those named by the case. While selecting such controls we need to be aware that these controls are closely matched to the cases on important characteristics and we may inadvertently have matched the cases and the controls on the exposure of interest by selecting them. To introduce some level of randomness in selecting these types of controls, we should obtain the name of more than one friend or colleague and select the actual control to be interviewed at random. In a study of childhood leukemia in Northern California, Ma et al. (23) randomly selected two controls for each case, one from computerized records of birth registries and the other from a list of friends provided by the families of cases. Both of these control groups were compared with a third control group whose selection was exactly population based with no attrition or data collection problems. The third group was considered as the "ideal" control group. The study concluded "that friend controls may not be representative of the study population and that there may be systematic differences by ethnic group in analyses in which friend controls are used." However, the results from their controls selected through the birth records were similar to the "ideal" population-based controls.

3.3.5.5 *Hospital visitors.* The approach in these controls is to select controls from the visitors of other patients in the hospital where the patient is admitted. The aim is to have nondiseased controls that come from the same community as the cases. Advantages for these controls include their accessibility, the possibility of conducting face-to-face interviews, concurrent interviewing with the cases, cost efficiency, and high response rates (24). This type of control should be selected in countries and communities where visiting hospital patients is a strong social obligation and the culture encourages people to do so. In such countries, we may be able to capture a broad cross-section of the population from within the hospital. This type of control has been used effectively in case-control studies in Lebanon, the Philippines, Tunisia, and Greece (24–27). In Lebanon the idea was tested first under conditions of a civil war when interviewing in neighborhoods was nearly impossible and telephone connections were close to nonexistent (24). Hospital visitor controls can be a source of bias, however, if the exposures of interest influence hospital visitation. For example, a study with smoking as a variable of interest should not use hospital visitor controls since smokers are not encouraged to enter hospitals due to no-smoking policies.

3.3.5.6 *Accident victims.* The theoretical basis upon which accident victims are selected as controls is that accidents occur at random and as controls the group may be a random selection of the population. However, there may be some common lifestyle factors that characterize accident victims that make them different from the general population.

3.3.5.7 *Pedestrian controls.* Honkanen et al. (28) conducted a case-control study of injuries due to accidental falls in public places in Helsinki, Finland, and studied its relationship to blood alcohol levels. Their cases were defined as injuries due to accidental falls in adults 15 years of age and older, and occurring between 3 and 11PM (due to limitations of study resources). For controls they selected two pedestrians of the same gender at random by visiting the site of the accident of the case exactly one week after the mishap. The authors assumed that day of the week and accident location were related to the accidents as well as to the alcohol use. By selecting pedestrians, they also selected active members of the community who were at risk for such accidents. They reported that alcohol increases a pedestrian's risk of accidental fall at a stronger level of association than a driver's risk of traffic accidents. Although there is a clear justification and a well-defined system of selecting these pedestrian controls in this particular study, one should be warned of the use of controls selected in a haphazard manner from a pedestrian population, because of the potential for selection biases in a study where the hypothesis under consideration may not warrant selecting such controls.

3.4 SELECTION BIASES

3.4.1 Overview

We are concerned about selection biases because they may lead to misclassification of case-control status, which may compromise our estimates of exposure or treatment effect and prognosis. Our framework for a causal relationship could also be jeopardized.

As quoted earlier from Feinleib, the underlying principle for biases and in particular selection biases is that "The probability of selection on the basis of disease status is not independent of the probability of selection by exposure status" (1).

Over the years a number of selection biases have been described, including Berksonian bias, diagnostic bias, prevalence-incidence bias (as described earlier), and detection bias.

3.4.2 Berksonian or Admission (Referral) Bias

This selection bias has been described in hospital-based case-control studies. It results from differential rates of admission between the case disease and the control disease, as well as differential admission rates to the hospital of exposed and nonexposed persons. If we are investigating the relationship of coronary heart disease and hypertension as the risk factor and we select controls from other diseases that have a different probability of admission to the hospital than coronary heart disease, a Berksonian bias may result because hypertension (the exposure) has another independent probability of admission to the hospital. A classic example of such bias is the 1929 case-control study of cancer and tuberculosis based on autopsy material from Johns Hopkins Hospital by Raymond Pearl, who was one of Berkson's teachers. From about 7,500 hospital autopsies Pearl identified 816 cases who had a cancer; he compared them to 816 controls without cancer (29). At autopsy, 16.3 % of the controls and only 6.6% of the cases of cancer had tuberculosis. His findings were confirmed through a number of subgroup analyses. He inferred that there might be an "antagonism" between cancer and tuberculosis. Further studies including animal experiments did not confirm Pearl's observation. Reviews of the case material of autopsies at the Johns Hopkins Hospital revealed that these autopsies were more common in tuberculosis patients (a disease of high interest at the time) than in other conditions. Thus, the controls were highly biased since Pearl had selected a group of patients who had died with tuberculosis. One can assume that there were differential probabilities of admission to the autopsy pool whether the person had cancer or the control conditions and the exposure of interest (tuberculosis) had its own independent probability for being autopsied.

It is important to note that in addition to Berksonian bias, Pearl's study may have been the subject of other biases, including prevalence-incidence bias and survival bias. Considering that his cases included a mix of incident and prevalent (autopsy discovered) cases, it may be possible that tuberculosis improved survival or duration with the disease (this is not an improbable option since today such a therapeutic effect of tuberculin is used in oncology for certain cancers).

3.4.3 *Surveillance Bias*

This is more of a problem with conditions that have asymptomatic or milder forms. Issues include whether the cases and controls were under equal intensity of surveillance for the disease in the prediagnosis period and whether the exposure affected the degree of surveillance between the cases and controls. If women taking oral contraceptives are more likely than other women to examine their breasts regularly, or have them examined by a medical professional, we may bias our results toward a probability of detecting more of the disease in those exposed to oral contraceptives (30). For example, if smokers receive more frequent medical attention for pulmonary disease, then they may be identified with pulmonary disease even if no real relationship exists between their smoking and the disease (2).

3.4.4 *Latency Bias*

Latency bias occurs when our selection of cases is within the period of latency of the disease. This is a situation where our ability to find an association between disease and exposure is hampered because the cases have not had the full run of the period of latency to become diseased. Such a bias will lead to misclassification of subclinical cases as controls. This problem is more serious with cancers and other chronic diseases where the period of latency or incubation between exposure and disease onset may be as long as several decades. The potential for such biases to occur is real when we are assessing an exposure that has been introduced recently in human populations and is changing rapidly. For example, a case-control study of oral contraceptives and breast cancer need not be conducted except after at least a decade of the introduction of the drug since the median latency of breast cancer is over 15 years (31).

3.4.5 *Enrollment Bias*

Enrollment bias results when, in a specialized clinical database, cases are selected from a period of time where the cases are more severe and certain disease–exposure associations are stronger than if a more representative series of cases were selected. In a clinic that was managing patients with familial paroxysmal polyserositis, the first 79 chronological cases of the disease that presented to the clinic were compared to the last 79 sequential cases on a number of etiological characteristics. The earlier cases had significantly stronger family history and were found to have more amyloidosis (a complication of the disease) than the later cases. Such enrollment differentials were able to explain important differences in reported findings of familial paroxysmal polyserositis in clinical case series from different countries (31).

3.4.6 Avoiding Selection Bias

It is important to design strategies to ascertain and test for potential biases whenever and wherever the possibility of such bias exists. At times one can obtain a credible estimate of the impact of a bias by testing the possibility in a small subsample of the study population. The following are strategies one may use to deal with selection bias during selection and during analysis:

3.4.6.1 *During selection.* Some of the strategies that may be useful in dealing with selection bias during selection are listed below:

1. Use a similar process of selection of cases and controls. All of the criteria used for exclusions and inclusions should be the same for cases and controls.
2. Ensure a high response or participation rate for both cases and controls.
3. Collect or pool the data from multiple hospitals or use multiple disease groups for controls.
4. Compare the exposure estimates in the control group to data from surveys of exposure in the general population to assess the potential of selection bias as to the exposure in the study groups.
5. Have the case and control selection process done by others than the interviewers.

3.4.6.2 *During analysis.* Some of the strategies that may be useful in dealing with selection bias during analysis are listed below:

1. Stratify and/or adjust for degree of surveillance used in cases and controls over the period prior to diagnosis.
2. Stratify and/or adjust for certainty of diagnosis based on the diagnostic information that is available. If a relationship exists, then in the subgroup with the more definite cases one expects the higher or more extreme odds ratios for the association with exposure.
3. Stratify cases by date of onset or diagnosis and compare relative frequency of exposure across these strata.
4. Assess the strength of the association. It is unlikely that an association with a large odds ratio will result from a biased study.

5. Assess the dose response between exposure and outcome. It is assumed that if there is a clear dose–response relationship the association will not be due to a selection bias.

6. Estimate the extent to which the presumed bias may explain the observed results. We may be able to present a range of estimates between the maximum effect and the absence of any effect of the bias.

REFERENCES

1. Feinleib M. Biases and weak associations. *Prev Med*. 1987 Mar;16(2): 150-164.

2. Sackett DL. Bias in analytic research. *J Chron Dis*. 1979; 32:51-63.

3. Antunes CM, Strolley PD, Rosenshein NB et al. Endometrial cancer and estrogen use. Report of a large case-control study. *N Engl J Med*. 1979;300:9-13.

4. Fried LP, Pearson TA. The association of risk factors with arteriographically defined coronary artery disease: what is the appropriate control group? *Am J Epidemiol*. 1987;125:844-853.

5. Hiller R, Sperduto RD, Ederer F. Epidemiologic associations with nuclear, cortical, and posterior subcapsular cataracts. *Am J Epidemiol*. 1986;124: 916-925.

6. Tung KH, Goodman MT, Wu AH, et al. Reproductive factors and epithelial ovarian cancer risk by histologic type: a multiethnic case-control study. *Am J Epidemiol*. 2003;158:629-638.

7. Murphy EA. The normal and the perils of the sylleptic argument. *Perspect Biol Med*. 1972;15:566-582.

8. Murphy EA. The normal. *Am J Epidemiol*. 1973; 403-411.

9. Schlesselman JJ. *Case Control Studies*. New York: Oxford University Press; 1982.

10. Howe GR. Using dead controls to adjust for confounders in case-control studies. *Am J Epidemiol*. 2001;134:689-690.

11. Falbo GH, Buzzetti R, Cattaneo A. Homicide in children and adolescents: a case-control study in Recife, Brazil. *Bull WHO*. 2001;79(1):2-7.

12. De Vries F, de Vries C, Cooper C, Leufkens B, van Staa TP. Reanalysis of two studies with contrasting results on the association between statin use and fracture risk: the General Practice Research Database. *Int J Epidemiol*. 2006;35:1301-1308.

13. Sulheim S, Holme I, Ekeland A, Bahr R. Helmet use and risk of injuries in alpine skiers and snowboarders. *JAMA*. 2006;295:919-24.

14. Linet MS, Brookmeyer R. Use of cancer controls in case-control cancer studies. *Am J Epidemiol*. 1987;125:1-11.

15. Blanchard JF, Armenian HK, Friesen PP. Risk factors for abdominal aortic aneurysm: results of a case-control study. *Am J Epidemiol*. 2000; 151:575-583.

16. Khachadurian AK, Uthman SM, Armenian HK. Association of tendon xanthomas and corneal arcus with coronary heart disease in heterozygous familial hypercholesterolemia. World Congress of Cardiology, Moscow, June 1982.

17. Thompson DC, Rivara FP, Thompson RS. Effectiveness of bicycle safety helmets in preventing head injuries. A case-control study. *JAMA*. 1996;276:1968-1973.

18. Koch M, Hanson J, Raphael M. Follow-up of controls participating in case-control studies for cancer risk factors. *Int J Epidemiol*. 1990;19:877-880.

19. Moritz DJ, Kelsey JL, Grisso JA. Hospital controls versus community controls: differences in inferences regarding risk factors for hip fracture. *Am J Epidemiol*. 1997; 145:653-660.

20. Olson SH, Mignone L, Harlap S. Selection of control groups by using a commercial database and random digit dialing. *Am J Epidemiol*. 2000;152:585-592.

21. Olson SH, Kelsey JL, Pearson T, Levin B. Evaluation of random digit dialing as a method of control selection in case-control studies. *Am J Epidemiol*. 1992;135:210-222.

22. Shaw GL, Tucker MA, Kase RG, Hoover RN. Problems ascertaining friend controls in a case-control study of lung cancer. *Am J Epidemiol*. 1991;133:63-66

23. Ma X, Buffler PA, Layefski M, Does MB, Reynolds P. Control selection strategies in case-control studies of childhood diseases. *Am J Epidemiol*. 2004;159:915-921.

24. Armenian HK, Lakkis NG, Sibai AM, Halabi SS. Hospital visitors as controls. *Am J Epidemiol*. 1988;127:404-406.

25. Ngelangel C. Hospital visitor-companions as a source of controls for case-control studies in the Philippines. *Int J Epidemiol*. 1989;18 (Suppl 2): S50-S53.

26. Bastuji-Garin S, Turki H, Mokhtar I, et al. Possible relation of Tunisian pemphigus with traditional cosmetics: a multicenter case-control study. *Am J Epidemiol*. 2002;155:249-256.

27. Polychronopoulo A, Tzonou A, Hsieh C, et al. Reproductive variables, tobacco, ethanol, coffee and somatometry as risk factors for ovarian cancer. *Int J Cancer*. 1993;55:402-407.

28. Honkanen R, Ertama L, Kuosmanen P, et al. The role of alcohol in accidental falls. J Studies Alcohol. 1983;44:231-245.

29. Pearl R. Cancer and tuberculosis. *American Journal of Hygiene*. 1929;9: 97-159.

30. Skegg DCG. Potential for bias in case-control studies of oral contraceptives and breast cancer. *Am J Epidemiol*. 1988;127:205-212.

31. McPherson K, Coope PA, Vessey MP. Early oral contraceptive use and breast cancer: theoretical effects of latency. *J Epidemiol Community Health*. 1986;40:289-294.

32. Armenian HK. Enrollment bias in familial paroxysmal polyserositis. *J Chronic Dis*. 1983;36:209-212.

4

AVOIDING INFORMATION BIAS IN EXPOSURE ASSESSMENT

Haroutune K. Armenian

OUTLINE

This chapter aims to

1. distinguish between the effects of differential and nondifferential measurement error in exposure measurement in case-control studies;
2. present various methods and sources of information about exposure;
3. discuss some common forms of information bias; and
4. list various strategies that are used for controlling or minimizing information bias in case-control studies.

4.1 MEASURING THE ASSOCIATION

The previous chapter provided an overview on case and control selection and approaches that will allow us to avoid selection biases. The current chapter will take a similar approach with exposure measurement. The ultimate objective of both processes of selection of study population and assessment of exposure is to obtain an unbiased measure of association between the outcome (disease) and the suspected factors.

Depending on the study design and the process of selection of the cases and controls, we may use different measures of association. The simplest approach to assessing the association was practiced prior to the development of the odds ratio in 1951 by Cornfield (1). These early approaches consisted of calculating the relative frequencies of exposure in cases and controls and making a judgment on the basis of a statistical significance test. With the development of the relative risk as a measure of association, it became critical to formulate the odds ratio as a method of approximating relative risk in case-control studies. Here the odds of exposure in the cases are measured and compared in a ratio to the odds of exposure in the controls. When we are selecting our controls concurrently to the case incidence time—incidence density sampling—a relative incidence rate is our aim for the measure of association. For most case-control studies, an odds ratio provides an acceptable estimate of relative risk. Morabia et al. (2), using data from the South Wales nickel refinery workers cohort where the outcome of respiratory cancers is quite common, and in a series of nested case-control analyses in different subcohorts, were able to demonstrate that the "Relative Incidence Rate was adequately estimated by the odds ratio when controls were identified concurrently to case occurrence throughout the risk period. The Relative Risk was well approximated with the Odds Ratio when controls were a sample of the study base." For Morabia and colleagues, the empirical data support the theory that the case-control method provides valid estimates of these measures of association.

The effect of various case-based designs on the measurement of an association will be discussed in more detail in Chapter 5.

4.2 EXPOSURE MEASUREMENT

4.2.1 Overview

In case-control studies we should ensure that our individual measurements have as little variability as possible. However, in addition to methodological issues that may affect such measurements, one needs to be aware of administrative, study management, and operational procedures and steps that may lead to biased results. For example, obtaining informed consent is a requirement for almost every study. It necessitates a well-defined protocol and the process may be time consuming. If, in a certain case-control study, the exposed cases in particular are reluctant to give such consent—perhaps for some legal consideration—then our assessment of the association will be based on a biased sample of the cases.

Our discussion on measurement of exposure is very much affected by a number of specific questions that have been expressed in assessing observational epidemiological studies and in particular case-control studies.

These questions are given below:

1. How do different exposures interact?
2. Now that we have mapped the human genome, how do exposures interact with genetic factors?
3. How can we determine levels of exposure below which there are no effects? Any thresholds?
4. How does the effect of the exposure change over time in a population?
5. Are we able to detect small effects following exposure?

Correa et al. (3), in a review of 223 case-control studies in 1992, categorized six different types of exposures in these studies: lifestyle, occupational factors, environmental factors, dietary factors, reproductive factors, and use of medications. Much of the exposure data that they studied were used as reported by the respondent, but for a number of studies using specialized questionnaires—such as a food frequency questionnaire—responses were converted to some summary values of exposure. Thus, beyond simple and direct measurements of exposure through questionnaires, one may need to use more complex conversions of data to assess exposure, such as using job exposure matrices that incorporate not just simple job titles but also industry, duration, and processes involved. A number of algorithms and conversion tables have been developed to assist in the measurement of exposure. In a number of areas, such as nutritional and occupational epidemiology, standardized questionnaires and instruments will help in generating the type of data that will be easy to convert to some standard summary measures, as well as to compare results with similar case-control studies.

Our primary concern for exposure measurement is *validity*. What is the sensitivity of our measurement in identifying people who are truly exposed? How specific is our measurement in identifying the nonexposed? Thus, we want first to make sure that the measurement of exposure has as few false positives and false negatives as possible. A number of studies have compared documented and recalled histories of exposure. In one such study, de Gonzalez et al. (4) assessed agreement between medical X-ray histories obtained from interviews and from medical records in two case-control studies. "In both studies, substantial disagreement was found between the number of X-ray examinations reported in the interview and in the medical records." However, in these two studies, the errors seemed to be nondifferential since estimates of risk were similar regardless of which data were used.

Prior to embarking on a measurement of exposure in case-control studies, it is important to assess the biological underpinnings of the exposure–disease relationship. We can address such a concern by raising a number of questions:

1. What is the potential of the suspected exposure to cause pathological changes in animal species, in other diseases or conditions?
2. What is the natural history of this exposure and how does this exposure cause the disease?
3. What is the latency or the incubation period for the disease with this exposure?

A clear idea of the period of latency for the disease may allow a more focused search for the period for which we are looking for the etiological factor. Our data collection strategies will differ in a case-control study based on whether we are dealing with a period of latency of days or years.

We want to make sure that our measurements are done without bias, and in a case-control study, bias can occur when *the process of measuring the exposure is not independent from the case-control status.* As an example, recall bias may occur when the cases remember their exposure to a radiologic procedure in childhood better than the controls.

4.2.2 The Kappa Statistic

We also need to be concerned about the *reliability or variability* of the process of measuring exposure. We would like to compare one instrument with another and assess their agreement as to measurements made on the same group of persons. We use a variety of methods to assess such reliability, including measures of agreement between investigators, measures of correlation, and the Kappa statistic:

$$\frac{\text{Observed Agreement} - \text{Expected Agreement (by chance alone)}}{1 - \text{Expected Agreement}}$$

The Kappa statistic will provide us with an assessment of agreement that is free of the effect of expected agreement by chance.

Whenever we are embarking on a measurement of exposure, it is important to use instruments or procedures for such measurement that have already been tested for reliability. For example, to assess such activity in a case-control study of 988 incident cases of prostate cancer and 1,063 population controls, Friedenreich et al. (5) used a questionnaire that had been already tested for reliability with a reliability correlation of 0.74 for total lifetime activity. Besides the tested reliability of the instruments, such an approach that uses established data collection instruments allows for comparisons across several studies of the disease that have used similar instruments.

It is critical that the population being investigated provides us with as much variability of exposure as possible. If almost everyone is exposed, we will not be able to measure such an association in this particular population because the differences between cases and controls will be negligible. According to Wynder and Stellman (6),

if cases and controls are drawn from a population in which the range of exposures is narrow, then a study may yield little information about potential health effects. This may be one reason why an association between dietary fat and cancer has not been consistently observed in Western populations. Since the fat intake as a percent of total calories in the US general population varies little, only very large relative risks can be detected in (such) epidemiologic studies.

If every person in the population uses cellular telephones then exposure to such telephones cannot be studied as a general risk factor for accidents unless the hypothesis is further refined to make the research question more specific. For example, the study could compare frequency and mode of use of cellular telephones as a cause of accidents.

In case-control studies misclassification is more of a problem in our measurement of exposure than disease status or outcome measurement. Errors of exposure measurement may lead to misclassification and can be sizable if they are not addressed.

4.2.3 Random Errors

Random errors in measurement are *nondifferential* between cases and controls and do not change across these study groups. As a result of such errors, random redistribution of study subjects occurs and such errors attenuate the measure of association toward their null value or an odds ratio of one. Often, such random errors may mask the existence of the association that we are trying to demonstrate (*except when there is perfect correlation between measured and true values*). Fung and Howe (7) reviewed the effect of joint misclassification of confounding as well as risk factor upon the estimation of the association. They found that if we have misclassification of the confounder in a situation where the error of the measurement of the main variable is nondifferential, then we may have an odds ratio that is biased away from one.

4.2.4 Systematic Errors or Differential Errors

This type of errors of measurement may result in a biased estimate of our findings. In this situation the amount of error in the controls differs from the amount of error in the cases. In this type of biased estimation, the odds ratio may move in any direction depending on the type and effect of the bias. As stated previously, these are situations where there is lack of independence of the processes of gathering the exposure information and case-control status. If a case is more likely to recall exposure than a control or if we are more likely to gather positive exposure histories from the cases than from the controls, then we may get an overestimated odds ratio if there is a positive relationship between exposure and outcome of interest.

Sosenko and Gardner (8) reviewed misclassification error in three studies and reported that "odds ratio estimates are more likely to be substantially biased from exposure misclassification when case-control studies have either very high or very low exposure frequencies."

4.2.5 Exposure Assessment Characteristics

Exposure needs to be defined not just as a function of a valid definition but also with regard to the time period during which exposure occurs. This time period is dependent on the latency of the condition.

If we inquire about the exposure up to 10 years in the past, then we are assuming that the latent period between the exposure and the development of the disease can be as long as 10 years.

In addition to these conceptual considerations, collection and validation of exposure information may be difficult. At every step of exposure assessment we may have problems that will affect the validity and reliability of our estimates. Thus the processes of data collection and exposure measurement in case-control studies should be planned and implemented very carefully. The following is a list of characteristics to consider when dealing with exposure assessment:

History of the exposure
1. Duration of exposure
2. Amount and intensity of exposure
3. Time at which exposure started or took place

Type and classification of exposure
1. Category where the exposure is classified from past experience
2. Threat or desirability of exposure for the general public

Method of measurement
1. Biological, pathological, clinical tests
2. Available records
3. Interviews and questionnaires

Scale of measurement
1. Binary (categorical)
2. Ordered or ordinal (e.g. small, medium, large)
3. Discrete (count)
4. Continuous

Every case-control study embarking on exposure measurement needs to address this list of characteristics, but unfortunately many published studies do not provide much of this information. According to Correa et al. (3), "rarely is the relevant exposure period specified or mentioned in the analysis." We also need to review the implementation of these studies, considering each of their peculiarities. In a case-control study of hip fractures in the elderly, Kelsey et al. (9) described a series of problems that they had encountered in carrying out the study. Some of these issues included cognitive impairment in the elderly and how it was addressed by the use of proxy respondents, questionnaire construction, response rates, interview process, memory, access to study subjects, and institutional review boards. Many of these issues will be discussed in the following sections of this chapter; we also recommend that readers review some of the original reports from the literature.

A number of studies have researched discrepancies between various methods of assessing exposure measurement. For example, Lichtman et al. (10) studied a group of individuals who failed to lose weight even though they reported restricting their caloric intake to less than 1200 kcal per day. Following detailed studies of energy expenditure, actual energy intake for 14 days by indirect calorimetry and analysis of body composition, the authors concluded that these subjects underreported their actual food intake by an average of 47% and overreported their physical activity by an average of 51%.

4.3 INSTRUMENTS OF EXPOSURE MEASUREMENT

Over the past two decades, the impact of technology on the process of measuring exposure has been dramatic. Such changes as telecommunication and networking have allowed epidemiologists to rethink their instruments of exposure measurement. Currently, computer-assisted interviewing is becoming more of a standard. Although answering machines and response control technology limit access to interviewees for random digit dialing (RDD), the vast increase in cheaper personal cellular telephone ownership places a larger number of individuals directly accessible as candidates for RDD.

Following are some of the methods of measuring the exposure in a case-control study.

4.3.1 Questionnaire-Based Studies

The majority of case-control studies are highly dependent on well-designed and structured questionnaires. Correa et al. (3), reviewing 223 case-control studies, reported that 83% of them had used a questionnaire to collect exposure data. There are a number of characteristics that one needs to look for in developing and using a questionnaire. These include clarity of the forms and the language, the ability of the questionnaire to raise the questions in a standardized manner, the logical ordering of the questions, the length of the questionnaire, and the time it takes to complete. A questionnaire that takes more than an hour to complete may lead to fatigue, particularly with sick individuals, which may affect the validity and reliability of the data collected. As an instrument of data collection, the questionnaire is able to collect detailed data on a variety of exposures and covariates. One can assess the duration, extent, and details of mode of exposure through a questionnaire. This explains the popularity of the questionnaire as a data collection instrument and the elasticity it offers with regard to a variety of approaches. Questions need to be as neutral as possible and should not lead to biased responses that reflect the preferences of the investigator.

The questionnaire may be *structured* with standardized questions that define the various options for a response (close-ended) or they may be *unstructured*, with response options not predefined. These unstructured questionnaires are usually *open-ended* allowing for a description of options and events, some of which may not have been predicted by the investigators. As such, these unstructured questionnaires are very useful when we are exploring various etiological possibilities or when we have set our study as a "fishing expedition" of a disease of unknown etiology. In such a situation, the interviewer is given more leeway in probing for responses. Case investigations (Chapter 1) fall into this category of probing, with regard to why this case developed the disease. However, an open-ended and unstructured questionnaire can present some problems that we need to consider. With such questions, problems in data processing may result when we attempt to categorize and organize responses in a manner useful for analysis. In addition, open-ended questions may provide us with superfluous data.

As an instrument, the questionnaire helps to elicit information from the respondent. Between the time the individual is asked the question and the time a response is given, the individual has to grasp what is being asked, get the information from memory, and provide an answer. At each step a possibility exists that due to past experience or current interpretation of events in the past, the respondent may provide us with an answer that may not totally represent the truth regarding past exposure. Lapses of memory and confusion may be limited to the disease under consideration; these lapses may be worse in acute phases of a condition, for example, post operatively (9). Interviewers of cases should consider such potential problems.

4.3.1.1 *Computer-assisted interviewing.* The advantages of computers in conducting interviews are numerous. As systems they provide more flexibility and simplify the flow of the interview based on the responses of the individual. A computer can be programmed to allow specific probing with predesigned questions, as well as to show visual aids. The program can also conduct on-the-spot quality and consistency checks of the data collected. This method of interviewing has been shown to increase responses on sensitive questions because of the improved privacy of the respondent. van de Wijgert et al. (11) tested such a system in Zimbabwe to find out whether it presented similar advantages in a developing country environment. The majority (86%) of the women participating preferred the computer-assisted method to the interviewer method. Computer-assisted data collection methods have been found to facilitate questionnaire design and testing, as well as detailed data collection.

4.3.1.2 *Mail questionnaire.* This relatively inexpensive method has been used to collect information on exposure and other characteristics of cases and controls. It is an efficient approach and some persons find it easier to respond to a questionnaire than to discuss sensitive issues with an interviewer. The method allows more time for the individual respondent to think and answer with more assurance and it is free of the possibility of interviewer bias. Still, a number of problems may plague a data collection process based on mailed questionnaires, including low response rates (less than 60% response rate after 3 mailings in some studies), and dependence on a mail system that in some countries may not be efficient. In using the mailed questionnaire, we need to make sure that the sequence of responses to the questions is not of critical importance to the study, because some of the respondents may not follow the order in which the questions are asked. Clarity of the questionnaire text is of paramount importance in these studies if no interviewer is present to explain the question. A mailed questionnaire will also prevent us from making direct observations on the individual respondents and of their environment. These latter observations may be important to assess the emotional reactions elicited by the questions, as well as for looking at ancillary evidence of exposure or data on socioeconomic characteristics. Bahl et al. (12) reported a case-control study from Canada using a mailed questionnaire. To test the hypothesis of whether the use of antidepressant medications was associated with an increased risk for non-Hodgkin's lymphoma, they mailed questionnaires to 723 cases of the disease; 638 (88%) responded. They also mailed similar questionnaires to 2,446 controls without the disease, selected from a government registry: 1,930 (79%) responded. The authors could not detect any association in their analysis. In particular, duration or histories of use or individual types of antidepressant medications were not associated with non-Hodgkin's lymphoma risk.

A number of studies have experimented with various interventions that may improve response rates to mailed questionnaires. Spry et al. (13) conducted three controlled experiments testing the efficacy of a postcard or telephone prompt, a lottery, monetary incentives, and questionnaire length in the recruitment process of adult respondents. The postcard plus lottery was up to 54% effective in eliciting a response. The shorter questionnaire alone, and the lottery alone, did not increase response rates significantly, relative to the long form, while the monetary incentive increased the response rates significantly. In another experiment, Eaker et al. (14) tested three methods of questionnaire mailing procedures in Sweden. Of eight possible combinations, the one comprising preliminary notification, a short questionnaire, and no mention of telephone contact yielded the highest retrieval rate. Young age, male sex, and urban residence significantly lowered the retrieval rate. Many of these findings may be specific to the study environment or influenced by cultural differentials, as highlighted by study findings from Hoffman et al. (15). The authors conducted a controlled trial of the effect of length, incentives, and follow-up techniques on responses to a mailed questionnaire in Washington County, MD. The response rates were similar for the short and long questionnaire groups; the monetary incentive did not improve the frequency of response; and the second mailing of a questionnaire was significantly more effective than a postcard reminder in improving responses (23% vs. 10%). The authors recommend using marketing principles to determine which approaches will improve response rates for mailed questionnaires. Including a study-logo pen or pencil with the mailed questionnaires, White et al. (16) were able to increase response rates by 15 to 19% in an experiment where at random a pen was included in the mailed package.

4.3.1.3 *In-person interviewing.* This is accepted as the preferred approach for gathering information for most case-control studies. The advantages of in-person interviewing include the ability to make direct observations on the household and on the reactions of the individual respondent, and to provide a subjective assessment of the potential truthfulness of the respondent. Potential problems with this approach include problems and biases of the interviewers, and the lack of standardization in the conduct of interviews. If distances and security are important concerns for conducting in-person interviewing, then we may not be able to achieve high participation rates. This approach introduces an important source of variability because of the variety of environments where the interviews are conducted, or because of the presence of other family members or colleagues during the interview. A major source of variability with this method of data collection relates to the interviewer. For example, nonuniformity among interviewers in asking questions, as well as misrecording the collected data can be problematic.

4.3.1.4 *Telephone interviewing.* This method of collecting data is efficient and safe. Using the random digit dialing (RDD) approach to identify potential candidates for interviewing is sometimes the first step of the process. RDD is effective for a study in locating potential subjects who are not listed in telephone directories. In a Chicago study, 31% of eligible participants identified through RDD had unlisted telephone numbers (17). Since telephone interviewing involves a live interview by trained personnel, many of the problems with in-person interviewing also apply to telephone interviewing. As with mailed questionnaires, it is not possible to make direct observations during telephone interviewing or to show pictures or samples of material to validate exposure. The interviewer has little flexibility to use probes or visual aids. However, Beresford and Coker (18) mailed a pictorial display of pills in a case-control study of past hormone use to the interviewees prior to the telephone interview. The display more than doubled the number of women recalling the name and dose of their hormonal therapy. Telephone interviewing is less expensive than in-person interviewing— some estimate that for every successful interview, it will cost 50% less than the in-person interview (19)—and provides easier access to potential study subjects. In a comparison of results obtained from interviews conducted through RDD and from groups from the same area where the individuals responded to self-administered surveys through mailed questionnaires, Link et al. (20) were able to demonstrate what had been observed in previous research that self-administered surveys generally produce higher estimates than interview-administered surveys.

4.3.1.5 *Proxy informants.* These are used in a number of special situations. Classic examples include relatives of dead cases or controls or of participants with Alzheimer's or other dementing illnesses (21). If exposure data for the cases are collected through a proxy, while data for the controls are collected from individual study subjects, then differentials in the validity of the exposure information between cases and controls may lead to biased estimates of the association. A recommended approach is to interview proxy respondents for both the live control and the dead case. Korten et al. (22) studied the level of agreement between individual interviews with selected controls and informant proxy interviews for Alzheimer's disease, using the Kappa statistic to assess agreement. "Agreement was best for exposures involving lifestyle, medical interventions or disorders of more recent origin, and worst for exposures which involved judgments by the respondent" (21). In a case-control study of oral cancers, Greenberg et al. (23) compared 23 cases with interviews of surrogates with 113 cases that were interviewed in person. Cases interviewed through a surrogate had more advanced disease, were sicker, were less educated, smoked more, and consumed more hard liquor than the cases that were interviewed personally. Lyon et al. (24) compared responses to interviews of 163 index subjects to a similar number of next-of-kin proxy respondents. Nonspouse proxies misclassified exposures more than spouses, and cigarette use was the most accurately reported exposure, followed by alcohol, coffee, and foods. The authors concluded, "that misclassification by proxy respondents is a function of multiple factors including the type of exposures under study and the type of proxies available."

A number of approaches can be used to improve questionnaires and the process of interviewing. Following the development of the questionnaire we need to *pilot test* it under circumstances similar to the actual study situation and decide what changes should be made to its various elements. We need to test for word and sentence comprehension and develop various memory helpers to encourage respondents to retrieve information from memory. For critical exposure information one may use a number of different approaches to elicit a response in the same questionnaire. For example, to assess the length of time for the exposure, we may use different benchmarks in the life of the individual and try to determine whether the person was exposed during those benchmarks.

4.3.2 Record-Based Studies

Records are reliable sources for identifying cases as well as controls but may have substantial limitations for gathering exposure information unless the data are collected in a standardized manner from everyone involved. Thus, in a hospital, data collected routinely on every patient and on admission may be more standardized than data collected as part of clinical assessment by health professionals. Such routinely collected data in records are very useful to evaluate the characteristics of respondents and nonrespondents in our study since these are available for the investigator who is interested in reviewing such parameters. In some hospitals the data collected routinely upon admission may go beyond the sociodemographic and administrative information. For about four decades, for example, every patient admitted to the Roswell Park Memorial Institute in Buffalo, NY, filled out an extensive epidemiological questionnaire on various lifestyle and exposure characteristics prior to the establishment of a diagnosis. These questionnaires formed the basis for a number of case-control studies of cancers of various sites.

There is much variation among the validity of the information available in various types of records. In a case-control study, if we are able to obtain data on exposure from available records—particularly when the data on these records was registered at a time when the exposure was occurring—we will get a most valid and reliable source of information. However, these records may also have problems of clarity and often may not have the detailed relevant information on exposure that we need. When we are relying on recorded information, we need to develop a standardized abstract form to extract the exposure data on the cases and controls. This process of abstracting the data has its own risk of random as well as systematic errors.

Records are kept on individuals for a variety of purposes and each of these records could become a valuable source of information in a case-control study. At birth, data is registered in birth registries as well as hospital records with information on the mother and her potential exposures. Medical records, whether these are clinic- or hospital-based, contain information on a number of medical exposures. Medical insurance records provide some detail on the transactions of the individual with the health-care provider and the health-care system. Employment records may be a rich source of data on occupational exposures and lifestyles.

4.3.2.1 *Medical records.* These are a frequent source of exposure data. Problems with medical records may include incomplete data, and lack of reliability and validity (due to evolving procedures and multiple persons involved in the measurements). Data on various exposures such as smoking are usually recorded poorly unless they are collected in an obligatory manner as part of the routine admissions data collection process.

4.3.2.2 *Occupational records.* A number of special problems can occur with data collected from occupational records for measuring exposure. These may include incomplete information as to the period of exposure in an occupation, a wrong job classification, arbitrary assignment of a job title, or job title falsely or inappropriately coded. It is useful to check information from recorded sources with participant interviews or other sources such as insurance records.

4.3.3 Biological and Other Special Instruments

4.3.3.1 *Overview.* Biological measurements may be used in case-control studies (1) as a *marker for exposure*, for example, measuring blood lead as a marker for exposure to lead; (2) as a measure of genetic *susceptibility to the etiological factor*, for example, measuring G6PD levels to assess susceptibility to exposures that in the absence of this enzyme may cause a hemolytic crisis; and (3) as a *marker for changes in the individual* resulting from the exposure. An example of the latter situation is a small outbreak of gynecomastia in prepubertal children. Blood and urine hormonal measurements were made in cases and controls to assess whether there was exposure to estrogens (25). Correa et al. (3) list the following characteristics for a biological marker: "1. specificity to a given agent; 2. persistence or degradation over time in a manner that preserves the order of cumulative exposures of study subjects; 3. detectability with available practical, accurate, and reliable assays; and 4. having a small ratio of intrasubject to intersubject variation."

4.3.3.2 *Special measurements.* These involve assessment of biological parameters for individual cases and controls through some live measurement or specimen collection process or collection of data on some environmental characteristic that may affect the development of the outcome in these individuals. One has to note that such measures may give a biased estimate of the association if measurements are made following the development of the disease rather than before, and thus subject to cross-sectional bias. Such a problem was faced by Beane Freeman et al. (26) in their case-control study of toenail arsenic content and cutaneous melanoma in Iowa. They studied arsenic concentrations in toenail clippings from 368 cutaneous melanoma cases and 373 colorectal cancer controls. They reported that elevated toenail arsenic concentrations increased the risk of melanoma (odds ratio = 2.1, 95% confidence interval: 1.4, 3.3). These authors made the assumption that toenail concentrations of arsenic reflect long-term exposure rather than recent changes that could be the result of the disease rather than its cause. Coultas et al. (27) assessed the reliability of questionnaire responses on lifetime exposure to tobacco smoke in the home in 149 adult nonsmokers, with information on exposure obtained twice in six months. They also compared these questionnaire results with urinary cotinine levels within 24 hours of the interview. There was a high level of agreement of parental smoking histories obtained six months apart but the urinary cotinine levels correlated only modestly with the reported exposures on the questionnaires.

4.3.3.3 *Specimen banks.* A number of case-control studies looking at the relationship of the role of biological parameters to the incidence of disease have been marred in the past by cross-sectional biases. In these studies the specimen collection was usually conducted following the development of the disease and it was unclear whether the changes observed in these biological parameters were etiologically related to the disease or were the result of the disease. To prevent such a cross-sectional or prevalence bias, longitudinal studies were initiated where the data samples were collected from the base population prior to the development of the disease and analyses were based on nested case-control studies. Specimen from the incident cases collected previously would be compared with similarly collected specimen from controls with no disease upon follow-up selected from the base population. Specimen banks have been developed to address a variety of diseases including cancer, AIDS, cardiovascular and neurological conditions.

4.4 INFORMATION BIAS OR BIAS IN THE ESTIMATION OF EXPOSURE

A variety of biases have been described that may lead to misclassification of exposure if the data collection process is not independent from the case-control status. These biases are discussed in the following sections.

4.4.1 Nonresponse Bias

This will occur if cases and controls have differential response rates to exposure information and we may be forced to use surrogate sources of information for missing data. Thus, we may observe differences between cases and controls in exposure rates, not because these differences are real but because the validity and reliability of the sources of data for cases and controls are significantly different. In a comparison of the characteristics of respondents and nonrespondents from a case-control study of breast cancer in younger women, Madigan et al. (28) reported a number of differences between the two study groups, some of which were related to the study hypotheses. However, "comparisons of crude and simulated relative risks using available nonrespondents' data generally showed a low impact of non-response on relative risks in this study." In a study of nonrespondents to self-administered questionnaires in Japan, Iwasaki et al. (29) reported that compared to nonparticipants, participants tended to be older, less educated, engaged in a different set of professions, smoked less, and had healthier dietary habits. Nonresponse may be more of a problem for mailed questionnaires than for in-person interviewing. Coogan and Rosenberg (30) tested whether a small financial incentive will alter case and control participation rates in an ongoing study of colorectal cancer. They concluded that, " among controls, a small monetary incentive appears to promote a feeling of goodwill toward the research. It does not seem to have an equivalent effect among cases, and in the worst case it may insult or annoy some cases who may otherwise have participated."

4.4.2 Recall Bias

As mentioned previously, cases may recall certain events better than controls or they may be more careful in their responses about exposure than controls and these differences may affect our estimates of the association between the outcome and the exposure (31). Also, if there is a case of the disease in the family, other family members may provide information about exposure thought to be related to the disease. Thus differential recall between cases and controls may result in a biased estimate of the association. Gibbons et al. (32) compared mothers' responses to a number of questions collected prospectively, to the same questions answered by the same mothers six weeks following the occurrence of sudden infant death syndrome in their offspring. The comparison was based on 27 cases and 25 controls and the Kappa statistic was used for assessing agreement. There was good agreement on demographic factors, maternal obstetric history, parental smoking, and infant feeding practices. Case mother reports regarding family history of disease and infant bedding were more discrepant. Houts et al. (33) compared 189 persons with cancer with their same-sex cancer-free siblings closest to them in age. Siblings with cancer had significantly higher reports of activities of daily living, nutrition, and emotional problems, and a significantly lower rate of family problems compared to the cancer-free siblings. Female and younger patients with cancer tended to report more problems than their siblings without cancer. In a review of the literature, Coughlin (34) has highlighted that recall bias is related to the characteristics of the exposure of interest and of the respondents. Interviewing technique, the design of questionnaire, and the motivation of the respondent may all lead to such biases.

The effect of such differential recall needs to be viewed, however, within the context of the particular case-control study, since factors such as the exposure in the study population may affect our estimates of the misclassification. Hopwood and Guidotti (35) reinterviewed 22 persons exposed to fumes containing nitric acid six months following a first interview that was conducted within 24 hours of the incident. More symptoms were reported in retrospect as occurring at exposure than in the original interview. Drews and Greenland (36) conducted a number of analyses and suggested that sometimes "even large differences in accuracy may have a minor impact on the results of the study. Study results may be particularly resistant to differences in the sensitivity of recall when the prevalence of exposure is low". Norell et al. (37) compared results obtained from a structured interview about lifetime oral contraceptive (OC) use with prescription records from a community-based sample of 427 women. Interview data and pharmacy records showed a high level of agreement for any OC use, current use, time since first and last use, and total duration of use. It is very rare to have such validation of exposure information from a source other than interview, and in particular from recorded information (38).

4.4.3 Interviewer Bias

This type of bias may occur when the interviewer favors a certain response differentially and unconsciously over another between the cases and controls, leading to misclassification. Such bias can also be generated when interviewers are aware of case-control status and may try to obtain information about exposure with more intensity from cases than from controls. Variability in approaches may lead us to inappropriate inferences. We expect interviewers to be tactful, careful, sensitive, polite, accurate, adaptable, interested, honest, and perseverant (39). One will need to go beyond the ideal to fulfill these criteria and most interviewers try to get as close as possible to this level. Appropriate training of interviewers and monitoring of the interviewing process could potentially control much of this type of bias.

4.5 MEANS OF CONTROLLING MEASUREMENT ERROR

In dealing with measurement error one may try to control such errors, minimize them, or measure the error. The latter approach is used to make the appropriate corrections in our estimates of association or risk during our analysis. No amount, however, of data handling, controlling for errors, and analytic procedures will replace the need to obtain the most valid information possible when we are measuring exposure. Our study design, our data collection instruments, and our procedures can make the difference between a good study and one that is burdened by innumerable problems and biases.

We may minimize these errors at the *design and organization* phase of the case-control study, ensuring that the appropriate guidelines are followed. We may also do a number of *pretests* of the study to correct any errors that may occur during the data gathering process. Other strategies to minimize such errors include spending much targeted effort on *interviewer training* and also the use of *multiple data sources* to validate the findings in at least a random subgroup of the study population.

We should begin by trying to minimize the nondifferential error before we try to quantify, measure, or estimate it. There are a number of strategies and measures one can use, which we list in the following sections.

4.5.1 Using Tested, Validated Instruments and Measures

1. Use questions that are tested and validated in other studies.
2. Provide in the questionnaire appropriate response options with categories that are mutually exclusive and exhaustive.

3. Use multiple measures of exposure to help improve the precision of our assessment of exposure.

4. Introduce in the questionnaire other exposures that are known not to be of etiologic significance but that sound intuitively as plausible to be associated with the disease (31) to deal with suspected recall bias, whereby cases may have a higher probability of remembering exposure than controls. Check whether these other variables are selected by the cases as often as the study exposure. If we are testing a certain drug X as a cause for congenital defects then we may also introduce in the questionnaire questions about the use of drugs Y and Z that are known not to cause such congenital defects.

5. Ask the respondent directly to identify which exposure they think causes the disease at the end of the interview to check for other respondent or interviewee biases.

6. Assess exposure as a multidimensional measurement by collecting data on its intensity, duration, and timing. Other details about the exposure that may play a critical role include first and last exposure time, and concurrent exposure to other agents that may interact with the exposure of interest.

4.5.2 Improvement of Data Collection Procedures

1. Conduct a pilot study. Such a study of the instruments and the procedures that are to be used needs to be conducted in the most realistic sample of potential candidates for study subjects and in an environment that tries to mimic study conditions.

2. Develop an interviewer's manual that explains clearly all the standard steps and procedures for the study and addresses potential problems and questions to be raised.

3. Consider using computer-assisted interviewing or data collection, if applicable, to improve standardization and minimize interviewer bias.

4. Conceal case-control status from the interviewers to prevent personal biases about an association between exposure and outcome to avoid influencing the data collection process.

5. Train interviewers uniformly. Such training should take into consideration all the possible biases that may occur in a study.

6. Apply quality control techniques to the interviewing process. Edwards et al. (40) used a system of audiotaping all interviews and coding a sample of these according to interviewer behaviors as to appropriateness in a large case-control study of colon cancer. The authors showed "that 94.2% of all questions were

asked in the same manner by all interviewers and that 89.5% of all probing behaviors were appropriate." These authors, using simulations, estimated that interviewer variability can drop study power from 84% to 56% and that the odds ratios could be biased downward from 1.8 to 1.3.

7. Use questions and techniques that increase memory retrieval like linking the questions to major events in the life of the interviewee.

8. Test for differential recall (31).

9. Interview cases and controls concurrently. This can prevent short-term changes such as seasonal variation from influencing the results. It is also possible that the staff involved in data collection may change over time; thus, case-control differences may reflect actual biases and differences involved in the data collection process through time. Concurrent interviewing will help minimize this. Concurrent data collection is also important for testing biological samples. Such samples should never be tested in separate batches for cases and controls, since conditions of testing may change with time due to changes in calibration of instruments and intra- and interobserver variability.

4.5.3 Improvement and Check of Recorded Information

1. Test for completeness, validity, and reliability of information by checking data from other sources, such as the original recorder of the record.

2. Design and test the abstract form carefully.

3. Train the record abstractors and provide appropriate supervision.

4. Blind the abstractors. It is preferable that the abstractors of the records do not know the study hypothesis. Such knowledge may lead an abstractor to look more carefully in the records for exposure in some study subjects than others, based on personal biases about the hypothesis.

5. Identify the original purpose of recording the information. Was the data collected for administrative purposes or were there research objectives that applied more rigor to the data collection process? If descriptive information is not available regarding the purposes and method of the original data collection, try to locate some of the people involved with these records early in their history to understand the reasons behind the initiation of the recording as well as its shortcomings.

6. Select record abstractors who have some knowledgeable background and train them appropriately. It is always good practice

to keep the individual who is abstracting the information blinded as to case-control status. Providing the abstractor copies of the records that have masked identifiers of the individual and case-control status can achieve such blinding.

4.5.4 Assessment of Effect of Bias during Data Analysis

1. Compare the results from the controls with available data from other sources such as surveys and census records. Use *dual sources of responses* on a sample of study subjects, comparing the standard instrument with a more valid data source.
2. Conduct a by-interviewer analysis of the study hypothesis to ascertain whether differences occur in the results that can be accounted for by interviewer bias.
3. Conduct a *special substudy* to measure *differential recall*. Following an estimation of the size of the error, one may be able to correct the estimates of the odds ratio or provide a range of values within which the correct estimate of the odds ratio may fall.
4. Assess the magnitude of the effect of the bias of measurement of exposure. The key question is whether the suspected bias is able to explain the observed association. If the calculated odds ratio is large (>3), then it is unlikely that a bias will be able to account for all of the observed effect.
5. Evaluate the potential effect of the bias in all subgroups of the study. Does this bias affect all subgroups to a similar extent?
6. Do not treat absence of data as a negative response in the analysis. Although in medical records the probability that we are dealing with a negative response is higher when there are no recorded data on a variable, we cannot assume that when the record does not have information on smoking the individual is a nonsmoker.

The critical nature of exposure assessment for the validity of results from case-control studies forces us to scrutinize our methods of data collection very carefully. The necessity for valid and reliable measurements applies to all approaches of exposure assessment.

The past couple of decades have seen a number of innovations in communication technology such as the worldwide massive use of cellular telephones and the use of the Internet. These changes dictate that we innovate in our traditional approaches to communicating with our study subjects. However, the principles that underlie our efforts to obtain valid and reliable data—such as independence of the two processes of data collection and case-control selection—remain constant across all methods.

REFERENCES

1. Cornfield J. A method of estimating comparative rates from clinical data. Application to cancer of the lung, breast and cervix. *J Natl Can Inst.* 1951;11:1269-1275.

2. Morabia A, Have TT, Landis JR. Empirical evaluation of the influence of control selection schemes on relative risk estimation: the Welsh nickel workers study. *Occup Environ Med.* 1995;52:489-493.

3. Correa A, Stewart WF, Yeh HC, Santos-Burgoa C. Exposure measurement in case-control studies: reported methods and recommendations. *Epidemiol Rev.* 1994;16:18-32.

4. de Gonzalez AB, Ekbom A, Glass AG, et al. Comparison of documented and recalled histories of exposure to diagnostic X-rays in case-control studies of thyroid cancer. *Am J Epidemiol.* 2003; 157:652-663.

5. Friedenreich CM, McGregor SE, Courneya KS, Angyalfi SJ, Elliott FG. Case-control study of lifetime total physical activity and prostate cancer risk. *Am J Epidemiol.* 2004;159:740-749.

6. Wynder EL, Stellman SD. The "over-exposed" control group. *Am J Epidemiol.* 1992;135:459-461.

7. Fung KY, Howe GR. Methodological issues in case-control studies III: The effect of joint misclassification of risk factors and confounding factors upon estimation and power. *Int J Epidemiol.* 1984;13:366-370.

8. Sosenko JM, Gardner LB. Attribute frequency and misclassification bias. *J Chron Dis.* 1987;40:203-207.

9. Kelsey JL, O'Brien LA, Grisso JA, Hoffman S. Issues in carrying out epidemiologic research in the elderly. *Am J Epidemiol.* 1989;130:857-866.

10. Lichtman SW, Pisarska K, Berman ER, et al. Discrepancy between self-reported and actual caloric intake and exercise in obese subjects. *N Engl J Med.* 1992; 327:1893-1898.

11. van de Wijgert J, Padian N, Shiboski S, Turner C. Is audio computer-assisted self-interviewing a feasible method of surveying in Zimbabwe?*Int J Epidemiol.* 2000 Oct;29(5):885-890.

12. Bahl S, Cotterchio M, Kreiger N, Klar N. Antidepressant medication use and non-Hodgkin's lymphoma risk: no association. *Am J Epidemiol.* 2004;160: 566-575.

13. Spry VM, Hovell MF, Sallis JG, et al. Recruiting survey respondents to mailed surveys: controlled trials of incentives and prompts. *Am J Epidemiol.* 1989;130:166-172.

14. Eaker S, Bergstrom R, Bergstrom A, Adami HO, Nyren O. Response rate to mailed epidemiologic questionnaires: a population-based randomized trial of variations in design and mailing routes. *Am J Epidemiol.* 1989; 147: 74-82.

15. Hoffman SC, Burke AE, Helzlsouer KJ, Comstock GW. Controlled trial of the effect of length, incentives, and follow-up techniques on response to a mailed questionnaire. *Am J Epidemiol.* 1998; 148:1007-1011.

16. White E, Carney PA, Kolar AS. Increasing response to mailed questionnaires by including a pencil/pen. *Am J Epidemiol.* 2005;162:261-266

17. Orden SR, Dyer AR, Liu K, et al. Random Digit Dialing in Chicago CARDIA: comparison of individuals with unlisted and listed telephone numbers. *Am J Epidemiol.* 1992;135:697-709.

18. Beresford SAA, Coker AL. Pictorially assisted recall of past hormone use in case-control studies. *Am J Epidemiol*. 1989;130:202-205.

19. Link, MW, Battaglia MP, Frankel MR, Osborn L, Mokdad AH. Address-based versus Random-Digit-Dial surveys: comparison of key health and risk indicators. *Am J Epidemiol*. 2006;164:1019-1025.

20. Frey JH. Survey Research by telephone. Sage Library of Social Research volume 150., Beverly Hills, CA: Sage Publications; 1983, p.31.

21. Schoenberg B. Epidemiology of Alzheimer's disease and other dementing illnesses. *J Chron Dis*. 1986; 39:1095-104.

22. Korten AE, Jorm AF, Henderson AS, et al. Control-informant agreement on exposure history in case-control studies of Alzheimer's disease. *Int J Epidemiol*. 1992;21:1121-1131.

23. Greenberg RS, Liff JM, Gregory HR, Brockman JE . The use of interviews with surrogate respondents in a case-control study of oral cancer. *Yale J Biology Medicine*. 1986;59:497-504.

24. Lyon JL, Egger MJ, Robison LM, French TK, Gao R. Misclassification of exposure in a case-control study: the effects of different types of exposure and different proxy respondents in a study of pancreatic cancer. *Epidemiology*. 1992;3:223-231.

25. Kimball AM, Hamadeh R, Mahmood RA, Khalfan S, Muhsin A, Ghabrial F, et al. Gynaecomastia among children in Bahrain. *Lancet*. 1981;21;1(8221): 671-672.

26. Beane Freeman LE, Dennis LK, Lynch CF, et al. Toenail arsenic content and cutaneous melanoma in Iowa. *Am J Epidemiol*. 2004;160:679-687.

27. Coultas DB, Peake GT, Samet JM. Questionnaire assessment of lifetime and recent exposure to environmental tobacco smoke. *Am J Epidemiol*. 1989; 130:338-347.

28. Madigan MP, Troisi R, Potischman N, et al. Characteristics of respondents and non-respondents from a case-control study of breast cancer in younger women. *Int J Epidemiol*. 2000;29:793-798.

29. Iwasaki M, Otani T, Yamamoto S, et al. Background characteristics of basic health examination participants: the JPHC study baseline survey. *J Epidemiol*. 2003;13:216-225.

30. Coogan PF, Rosenberg L. Impact of a financial incentive on case and control participation in a telephone interview. *Am J Epidemiol*. 2004 Aug 1;160(3):295-298.

31. Raphael K. Recall bias: a proposal for assessment and control. *Int J Epidemiol*. 1987;16:167-170.

32. Gibbons LE, Ponsonby AL, Dwyer T. A comparison of prospective and retrospective responses on sudden infant death syndrome by case and control mothers. *Am J Epidemiol*. 1993;137:654-659.

33. Houts PS, Yasko JM, Simmonds MA, et al. A comparison of problems reported by persons with cancer and their same sex siblings. *J Clin Epidemiol*. 1988;41:875-881.

34. Coughlin SS. Recall bias in epidemiologic studies. *J Clin Epidemiol*. 1990;43:87-91.

35. Hopwood DG, Guidotti TL. Recall bias in exposed subjects following a toxic exposure incident. *Arch Environ Health*. 1988;43:234-237.

36. Drews CD, Greenland S. The impact of differential recall on the results of case-control studies. *Int J Epidemiol*. 1990;19:1107-1112.

37. Norell SE, Boethius G, Persson I. Oral contraceptive use: interview data versus pharmacy records. *Int J Epidemiol.* 1998;27:1033-1037.
38. Skegg DCG. Potential for bias in case-control studies of oral contraceptives and breast cancer. *Am J Epidemiol.* 1988;127:205-212.
39. Kelsey JL, Whittemore AS, Evans AS, Thompson WD. *Methods in Observational Epidemiology.* New York, Oxford: Oxford University Press; 1996: p. 374.
40. Edwards S, Slattery ML, Mori M, et al. Objective system for interviewer performance evaluation for use in epidemiologic studies. *Am J Epidemiol.* 1994;140:1020-1028.

5

ALTERNATIVE CASE-BASED DESIGNS

Haroutune K. Armenian and
Gayane Yenokyan

OUTLINE

5.1 MAKING THE APPROPRIATE INFERENCES

Our inferences in epidemiology are dependent on our ability to

- *find the appropriate comparison group.* In a case-control or other case-based design, cases with a certain outcome are compared to persons or situations where the outcome of interest is absent. The comparison group provides the reference for the level of exposure against which exposure level in cases is compared. The comparative approach allows us to deduce whether, on average, cases are more or less exposed than the group without the outcome.
- *relate the exposure to the outcome across a clearly defined time sequence, where exposure antedates outcome.* Case-control and

other case-based studies are especially vulnerable to this criterion. The designs described in this chapter address this important concern.

- *assess changes in the outcome as well as the exposure over time.* A case-control or a case-based design may be able to capitalize on these changes to study variability in the relationship between presumed exposure and outcome and to make inferences from such changes.
- *refer to a base population.* Beyond delimiting our ability to generalize to a group of people, the existence of such a base population in case-control and other case-based studies will allow us to choose an appropriate comparison group. If all the cases and the comparison group are selected from the same base cohort, the study is nested within the cohort. This is the approach in nested *case-control* and nested *case-cohort* study designs.

In the pages ahead, as we discuss the various alternative case-based designs, it is important to study these alternatives by configuring the approaches they use in addressing these inferential concerns.

5.2 CASE-CROSSOVER DESIGN

5.2.1 Overview

As presented in the first chapter, a *case series* is an important tool for clinical investigation since it represents an attempt to define the disease and explain some of its pathogenesis and other processes involved in its development. The case series is also useful to study survival and to relate survival to various characteristics or interventions. As we stated earlier, the case series may be useful as an inferential tool if we are able to do some internal comparisons. For example, by comparing 40 typhoid fever patients with a certain complication of the disease (enteric or intestinal perforation) to 80 other patients with typhoid fever without the complication, Hosoglu et al. (1) reported that a short duration of symptoms, inadequate antimicrobial therapy, male sex, and leukopenia were independent risk factors for enteric perforation in patients with typhoid fever.

In addition to the case series, other study designs are also based on groups of cases. In genetics (see Chapter 8), case-only designs have been used frequently. Case-crossover is one of such designs, where event and control information are derived from the cases. The basic idea is to compare a patient's antecedent experiences to illness with the experiences during a time when the patient was not ill. The information about several patients can be pulled to understand the role of exposure in developing the outcome, that is becoming a case. This method has been used for case investigation in clinical practice for many years. Allergologists, for example, when investigating determinants of atopic reactions, would systematically review case histories of exposures just prior to a patient's allergic reaction for unusual exposures and compare them to the patient's experiences during "normal times." In other situations one may ask why did a patient develop a particular disease at this point in time? What was different in the life of this patient in the period prior to the onset of this recent illness compared to the "normal" times that may explain the disease onset?

There are a number of variations of case-crossover design. The simplest form of case-crossover design is to study the same cases at two time points, once as cases and a second time as controls. The exposures antecedent to the two states are compared. A comparison of level of exposure between case times and control times allows us to understand the relative importance of the exposure in the etiology of the disease or case status. In order to make the comparison, the investigator needs to define a time period prior to the onset of the disease, the *case window*, when the risk of developing the disease might be highest due to the exposure. The exposure level during the case window is then compared to the exposure level in the *control window*, a randomly selected time period of the same length as the case window. Referring to the inferential concerns described in the beginning of this chapter, control windows provide the reference level of exposure in the absence of condition and become the comparison group against which the exposure in the case window is compared.

Malcolm Maclure first used the term case-crossover for this design in a situation where investigators wanted to assess the immediate determinants of the acute event of myocardial infarction (2). Based on the evidence of high frequency of myocardial infarctions during early morning hours, the investigators developed a hypothesis that the condition is triggered by activities immediately prior to its occurrence. Their challenge was to identify the appropriate controls for cases of myocardial infarction. Difficulties in the recruitment of healthy representatives of the population, the potential selection biases associated with hospital controls, and the need to select controls from the same population base as the cases caused them to consider using the cases themselves at a healthy antecedent point in time as their own controls.

5.2.2 When to Choose the Case-Crossover Design?

When is the use of case-crossover design warranted? There are several requirements for using the design to estimate the effect of a hypothesized agent or exposure on the outcome of interest. Since, in a case-crossover study, the same individual provides data about exposure at two time points, conditions with very long latency lasting, for example, for years may not be amenable to this method. Thus, the case-crossover design is useful to study *transient effects* and *acute events with a short latency.*

The success of the case-crossover design is dependent on the dual *variability of disease and exposure status* in the individual. If we do not have such variability we will not be able to make any comparisons. Thus, this design will not be useful in situations where the disease status is fixed, such as in genetic diseases, and/or where the exposure characteristic is fixed or invariant, such as blood groups.

The use of information from the same cases at two points in time is attractive to investigate precipitants of *acute events*, particularly in atopic conditions like asthma and a variety of allergies. For example, in 1974 we considered the design for the investigation of precipitants for attacks of familial paroxysmal polyserositis or familial Mediterranean fever. This is a genetic disease that affects people of Middle Eastern origin and is manifested by attacks of peritonitis and inflammation of other serous membranes that have an acute onset and last for about 48 to 72 hours. In between attacks, patients with the condition have no symptoms. Based on a variety of observations and findings, it was hypothesized that in addition to the genetic predisposition, certain environmental exposures precipitated the attacks of acute abdominal tenderness with fever (3). It was proposed that gathering data on patients about such potential exposures at two time points would help to identify some of these precipitants. Thus, the patients would be examined during an attack to gather data about exposures during a period of about three days prior to the attack, and for a similar control period, selected at random, at a time when the patient was free of the attacks for at least a week. The period of inquiry for exposures (exposure windows) was limited to three days since this was the assumed period of maximum latency for the precipitants to generate an attack. The latency was estimated from a study of the records of over a hundred patients with regular recording of the frequency of attacks. It was assumed that the latency for the attacks was shorter than the period of time between the two attacks that were closest in time.

Other diseases and conditions that have been studied using the case-crossover design include myocardial infarction (4,5), birth defects (6), injuries (7), health services quality assessment (8), morbidity and mortality due to air pollution (9), and HIV/AIDS (10). In all these cases the outcome of interest was a well-defined, acute event, with a clear-cut onset. These characteristics ensure that the case window—the period of time prior to the outcome when exposure is measured—can be defined unambiguously. Consequently, this improves recall in cases when exposure is self-reported and, in general, facilitates exposure measurement.

One of the major concerns hindering inference is the difficulty of establishing antecedence of exposure in case-based designs. Therefore, a clear definition of the outcome and, consequently, the exposure window prior to the outcome increases the possibility that the temporal relationship between the exposure and the outcome can be established.

For example, in a study of the role of anger in myocardial infarction, a 2-hour period before myocardial infarction was considered the case window (4). Patients were asked questions regarding the state of anger first focusing on a 2-hour period prior to the onset of symptoms, then on the same time period on the preceding day. Since for such an acute event as myocardial infarction the onset of symptoms can be determined with relative precision for most patients, the exposure information can be collected with higher validity and reliability than for other events.

Another study directly assessed test-retest reliability of self-reported exposure to risk factors of occupational acute hand injury among 29 subjects who were interviewed repeatedly up to 4 days after the initial interview (7). Reliability of information about the self-reported exposures in the month prior to injury varied from 0.84 to 0.99 as measured by the intraclass coefficient.

The second requirement of the design is that the exposure of interest or its effect on the disease or condition needs to be transient. The case-crossover design is akin to the *crossover trials* in drug trials where the same individuals will sequentially receive both alternatives of the treatment trial. In such a study each participant serves as his or her own control, making it the closest matched experiment possible. Such a crossover trial may be randomized whereby individuals will be allocated randomly to one of the arms of the trial and then shifted to the other alternative, giving enough time and opportunity for therapeutic response. This approach, however, assumes that the effect of each of the therapeutic agents is immediate and not longlasting.

Further, to identify the role of exposure in developing the outcome of interest, there should be *variability in outcome state*. For each case patient the investigators should be able to define time periods in the past and/or in the future when the outcome of interest was absent. These times will define the potential control windows or reference times. So far we have pointed to having just one control window for each case window. Other variations of the case-crossover design include increasing the number of control windows up to the point of including the total case history or including control windows following the case window, especially for recurrent conditions (i.e., bidirectional sampling of control windows). Exposure level during control times can be measured directly or estimated using the usual frequency method suggested by Maclure (2). We will refer to this method in the Section on Analysis of Case-Crossover Data.

Finally, to compare case and control windows to identify potential etiological agents in developing the outcome of interest, there should be *variability in exposure state*. If a patient had been exposed to the proposed agent at all times, including the case window, it will not be possible to attribute development of the outcome under consideration to that exposure. Only patients in whom exposure during case and control windows potentially differ provide the data toward estimating the effect of the exposure on the outcome.

5.2.3 *Highlights of the Case-Crossover Design*

The salient points of the case-crossover design are listed below. This method is useful to *identify precipitating causes* of the outcome that occur close to the development of the condition.

1. Since each subject serves as his or her own control, the method *minimizes between-person confounding* by factors that do not vary in time (time-fixed factors). However, one must consider controlling for time-varying confounders, factors that change in time and may affect the relationship between the outcome and the presumed etiological agent. Confounding is discussed in more detail in the Section on Confounding and Effect Modification in Case-Crossover Studies.

2. Problems relating to control selection are absent from case-crossover studies because selection of a comparison group that is representative of the same base population is not a concern. Thus, issues of *selection bias* are minimized.

3. Following every exposure one may identify an *effect period* during which one expects the onset of the disease or condition. Thus, after each exposure the probability exists for the disease to develop in the individual. This probability is influenced by other factors that interact with the presumed exposure, one explanation for why an event of disease does not occur each time one is exposed to the presumed agent.

4. In a case-crossover study it is critical to understand the *latency period* for the development of the disease or condition. It is this length of time between exposure and onset of the disease that is used as a time frame for which one will try to identify exposures.

Thus, for transient effects, this period may be short and expressed in hours or days, while for some chronic illnesses the data collection process may require a period that spans several years. When there is little or no antecedent knowledge about the latency of the disease, one may decide to test various lengths of time for such a period. If an association with a particular exposure is identified, the length of the period of case-time when the odds ratio is maximized will be equivalent to the median latent period of the disease (11). For more on incorporating this estimation into data analysis see Mittleman et al. (4).

5. A common problem that may occur in a case-crossover study is that *temporal trends in exposure* may occur. In such situations associations between exposure and case development will be biased and will not reflect the true effect. For example, in a study of the effect of folic acid antagonist medications on cardiovascular birth defects the authors compared exposure during the second and third lunar month of pregnancy (case window) to the exposure during two months preceding the last menstrual period (control window). This analysis showed no association between folic acid antagonists and development of cardiovascular birth defects. However, the relationship has been shown previously in a case-control study with mothers of noncardiovascular defects as controls. The authors hypothesized that the conflicting results might be due to time trends in exposure: use of the folic acid antagonist often decreases with pregnancy (time trend in exposure). If this argument is true, it would result in higher probability of exposure in the control window compared to the probability of exposure in the case window. Therefore, one would expect that the estimated case-crossover odds ratio is an underestimate. Consequently, the investigators changed the definition of control window to fourth and fifth lunar months of pregnancy. In this case the exposure during the control window (fourth and fifth months of pregnancy) was similar to the exposure during the case window (second and third months of pregnancy). As a result, the authors obtained an odds ratio close to the one identified by the case-control study (6).

6. This study demonstrates the importance of selecting control windows to represent the referent exposure for the case window. Some authors suggest including several control windows, some prior to and some following the case window, to identify and correct for the time trends in exposure. For a further and more technical discussion see Navidi (12). One can enjoy the flexibility

of selecting multiple control windows when dealing with episodic conditions. However, if the outcome of interest is a chronic disease, one needs to exert more care in selecting controls after the disease. The control windows after the case windows might represent changes that result from experiencing the event.

7. As an efficient design, the case-crossover method *allows investigation of a condition when, due to limited resources or other considerations, one may not be able to recruit separate controls*; or one may be dealing with such a specialized referral pattern for the cases that it may not be possible to identify a base population for the cases from which one may select controls.

5.2.4 *Potential Problems and Challenges*

Case-crossover studies pose some challenges and problems, which are listed below:

Carryover and period effects. Problems may arise when dealing with long latency periods, and the effect of one exposure period may overlap with another period of exposure.

Patient selection. Although it is unlikely that selection bias will occur in case-crossover studies, it is possible that the cases who are included in the investigation and interviewed may be a select subgroup of the cases that have either extremes of exposure (such as people who abstain from noxious habits or those who have been heavily exposed) and are interested in the study. Under such circumstances the cases may remember more intensely the exposures around the disease period compared to control periods. The potential for this factor to act as a source of selection bias is minimal, as most case-crossover studies are concerned with transient effects rather than lifelong exposures.

Latency effects. It is important to leave a "washout" period between the case and control windows that are longer than the period of maximum latency for the development of the outcome condition. It is also important to ensure that the control period does not overlap with the latency period of the effect of exposure on the outcome.

Information bias. As the same individual is providing a history of exposure for the case and control periods, there may be lapses of memory that may create a differential reporting pattern between the two periods. Depending on the timing, sequence, and length of time between case and control periods, one may end up with differences in actual exposure information between case and control periods that may be artifactual rather than real. However, some exposures may be more resistant to such frailties of memory, and the exposure information collected at two time points should be validated in a sub sample.

An investigator who selects the control period systematically prior to the case period could bias the results when dealing with "naturally" occurring time trends for the exposure in the population. Estimating and taking into account such an effect of time trends in the analysis may be achieved by conducting a *case-time-control design*, where one adjusts for the time trends of exposure measured in a control group. In this situation, much of the efficiency of a case-crossover design— compared to the case-control method—will be lost since one is obligated to develop a control group.

For example, Schneider et al. tested the hypothesis of potential triggering factors for T-cell homeostasis failure (TCHF), a sudden decline in the CD3+ cell count levels occurring approximately 1.75 years prior to the onset of AIDS among HIV-positive individuals (10). The following exposures were investigated: sexual behavior (the number of male partners), use of recreational drugs (marijuana/hashish, poppers, cocaine), and reported STDs (gonorrhea, syphilis, genital warts). Since the exact time of T-cell failure was unknown, the investigators estimated this time point between the two semiannual visits. The case visit was defined as the study visit immediately prior to the estimated point of T-cell failure. Control visits were defined as 1, 2, 3, 4, and 5 visits prior to the case window. The case-crossover analysis estimated the statistically significant protective effect for recreational drug use.

Additional analysis revealed a downward exposure time trend in the use of recreational drugs during the control periods among the cases. An analogous time trend was revealed in the control group that consisted of HIV-infected men who did not have AIDS and had no evidence of T-cell homeostasis failure. These controls were used in a *case-time-control analysis* (see Figure 5.1). For every control, a case-matched visit was defined, which coincided with the estimated point of T-cell failure in cases. Up to five visits prior to the case-matched visit provided information on exposure among the controls.

Temporal trends. Case-time-control analysis allows estimating and correcting for time trends in exposure. The information on the time trend in exposure comes from the control group. In particular, Schneider et al. calculated the odds ratio of exposure by comparing the case-matched visit to one of the control visits. This measure reflects the change in exposure in controls over time. Consequently, the case-crossover odds ratio is divided by the odds ratio measuring the temporal trend in exposure to arrive at the corrected, case-time-control odds ratio. In this study,

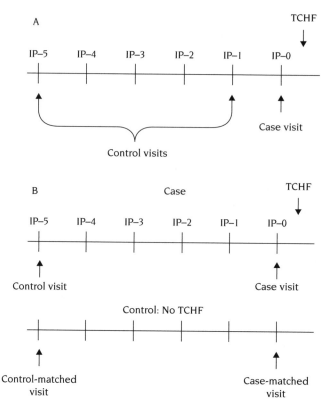

Figure 5.1. Case-Crossover (A) and Case-Time-Control (B) Designs
Adapted from Schneider et al. (10).

after correcting for the time trend the estimates were not statistically significant, although still below one (10).

5.2.5 Analysis of Case-Crossover Data

As mentioned earlier, control windows in a case-crossover study represent the referent exposure level, or the exposure level under the null hypothesis, to be compared to the exposure level in the case window. The same mechanism is used in a traditional case-control study where exposure frequency in controls serves as an estimate of the exposure level in the base population.

Selecting between the two main approaches to the analysis of case-crossover data depends on the method used to estimate the referent exposure level. The first is the method proposed by Maclure in his original paper (2). It is called "usual frequency" approach and is based on the concept of person-time and its apportioning into exposed and unexposed person-time. In this case we derive the estimate of incidence rate ratio representing the ratio of rate of outcome occurrence during the exposed and the unexposed person-time. The second approach is based on matched analysis. It provides an estimate of the incidence rate ratio by comparing the difference between two ratios: (1) the number of exposed case windows to the number of unexposed control windows, and (2) the number of unexposed case windows to the number of exposed control windows. Patients who were exposed during both case and control windows as well as patients who were unexposed at both times represent *concordant sets* and do not contribute to the estimate of the incidence rate ratio. In the next section both methods will be discussed in greater detail.

5.2.5.1 *Usual frequency analysis.* Usual frequency method is based on the assumption that each study participant in a case-crossover study represents a follow-up time, which is sampled to obtain case and control windows. The total follow-up time is divided into exposed and unexposed person-time. To obtain the estimates of exposed and unexposed person-time, patients are asked about the usual frequency of exposure during a significant amount of time, such as a year or a month prior to the development of the disease. Exposed person-time is obtained by multiplying the usual frequency by the duration of the hypothesized hazard period. For example, in a study of heavy physical activity and development of FMF attacks, if a patient usually engages in heavy physical activity once a week and if the duration of hypothesized hazard period is 2 days, then in a month prior to an FMF attack, the patients will be exposed for a total of 4×2 days = 8 days. The unexposed person-time is attained by subtracting exposed person-time from the total person-time. In our example, we estimated the patient will be exposed 8 days out of 30 (one month), while she will be unexposed for 22 days in a month. For similar examples see Maclure (2).

The case event (in our example, FMF attack) can be either exposed or unexposed and is classified as exposed if the patient reports being exposed within the case window (two days prior to FMF attack in the example above). If exposure occurred more than two days before the attack, the latter is counted as an unexposed event.

Based on the information on usual frequency as well as exposure within case windows, the analyst can construct a 2×2 table that will summarize the exposure–outcome relationship for each patient.

Consider the following two patients. Patient 1 engages in heavy physical activity once a week and reported an FMF attack within less than two days after she was last physically active. Patient 2, on the other hand, is engaged in heavy physical activity twice a month and

Patient 1

	Exposure within case window	
	Yes	No
FMF attack	1	0
Person-days	8	22

Patient 2

	Exposure within case window	
	Yes	No
FMF attack	0	1
Person-days	4	26

Figure 5.2. Exposure–Outcome Relationship

reported no exposure within two days of his FMF attack. Applying the usual frequency approach, Patient 1 was exposed for 8 days and unexposed for 22 days within the last month. In her FMF attack, the case event is considered exposed. For Patient 2 we calculate $2 \times 2 = 4$ days of exposure and 26 days of no exposure. His FMF attack is considered unexposed.

We can therefore construct the 2×2 table (Figure 5.2) based on the above information.

An estimate of incidence rate ratio can be calculated for each table. Since studies enroll more than one patient, we must combine all of the individual incidence ratio estimates into one pooled estimate. For that the Mantel-Haenszel estimator and its variance have been shown to be the best choice. The estimate of relative rate and the variance of the log of the relative rate are given by the formulas given below:

$$RR_{MH} = \frac{\sum_i \dfrac{A_{1i} \times N_{0i}}{N_{+i}}}{\sum_i \dfrac{A_{0i} \times N_{1i}}{N_{+i}}} \qquad var[logRR_{MH}] = \frac{\sum_i \dfrac{(A_{1i} + A_{0i}) \times N_{1i} \times N_{0i}}{(N_{+i})^2}}{\left(\sum_i \dfrac{A_{1i} \times N_{0i}}{N_{+i}}\right) \times \left(\sum_i \dfrac{A_{0i} \times N_{1i}}{N_{+i}}\right)}$$

where RR_{MH} is the Mantel-Haenszel estimator of the relative rate, A_1 and A_0 are the numbers of exposed and unexposed cases respectively, N_1 and N_0 represent the exposed and unexposed person-time respectively, and N_+ is the total person-time. Index i refers to each patient in the study.

Using the data of our 2 patients and the formula above, we get

$$RR_{MH} = \frac{\dfrac{1 \times 22}{30} + \dfrac{0 \times 26}{30}}{\dfrac{0 \times 8}{30} + \dfrac{1 \times 4}{30}} = 5.5$$

The usual frequency approach is fairly common in case-crossover studies. Sorock et al. used this method to obtain exposure information during control time by asking subjects in occupational health clinics to estimate their average frequency and duration of exposure to each of the hypothesized work-related triggers in the past month (7).

5.2.5.2 *Matched analysis.* A simpler iteration of the analysis of data in a case-crossover study uses a standard matched case-control approach with an odds ratio estimate from the ratio of discordant pairs. In a matched case-control study the pairs of matched cases and controls with only one exposed study participant contribute to the data analysis (see Chapter 6). The difference is that in a case-crossover study we will have discordance in exposure between case and control windows, rather than between matched case and control individuals. For example, in the case-crossover analysis of the birth defect data the subjects who were exposed to folic acid antagonists either during second and third lunar months of pregnancy ("case window") or during two months preceding the last menstrual period ("control window") contributed to the estimation of the odds ratio.

The study data are presented in Table 5.1 (6).

The odds ratio is equal to the ratio of the number of pairs where patients were only exposed during the case window (15 such pairs from Table 5.1) to the number of pairs where patients were only exposed during the control window (again 15 such pairs). The analysis yielded the estimated odds ratio of 1.0, suggesting no role for folic acid antagonists in development of cardiovascular birth defects (6).

The concept of matched analysis can be easily generalized to using more than one control window per patient. In this case, methods for 1:M matched case-control studies are applicable. For a detailed explanation and derivation of the method see Breslow and Day (13). Matched analysis will be also covered in Chapter 6.

5.2.6 Confounding and Effect Modification in Case-Crossover Studies

Since in case-crossover studies exposure information during case and control windows is derived from the same patient, an important advantage of

Table 5.1. Matched Analysis of Exposure Data

		Case Window	
		Exposed	Unexposed
Control Window	Exposed	48	15
	Unexposed	15	3,792

the design is that the data are matched on all patient-level characteristics, which do not vary in time. This means that there is no variability between case and control windows with respect to all potential confounders that are fixed in time (*time-invariant confounders*). If, however, the researcher suspects the presence of confounders that vary with time (*time-varying confounders*), he or she needs to adjust for these factors.

How can time-varying confounding occur in case-crossover studies? If the outcome event is believed to be affected by several triggers and if the triggers are correlated within the study, then the effect of one is likely to be confounded by the other. For instance, as discussed by Maclure in the study of triggers of myocardial infarction, several factors are believed to influence the risk of myocardial infarction, such as coffee drinking and sexual activity. If the patients are more likely to drink coffee after sexual activity, there will be an association between sexual activity (potential confounder) and coffee drinking (the exposure) in the data. Moreover, if both factors indeed alter the risk of myocardial infarction, sexual activity will act as within-person, time-varying confounder, and the effect of coffee drinking on myocardial infarction will be confounded by sexual activity (2). Analogously, in a study of triggers of FMF episodes, it is possible that the patients reduce the level of their physical activity during menstrual periods. Therefore, physical activity and menstruation will be negatively correlated. Since both are hypothesized to affect the risk of developing FMF attacks, the odds ratio associated with physical activity will be confounded by menstruation. One approach for addressing such confounding is to collect information on the amount of time of co-occurrence of the correlated exposures and to control the confounding by further stratification assuming that sufficient data will be collected in each stratum to estimate the effect of the exposure (2, p.149). Conditional logistic regression (to be discussed in Chapter 6) can also be used to adjust for within-person time-dependent confounding (14).

Effect modification can also occur in case-crossover studies. The effect of a trigger under consideration might vary in the presence of, or across levels of, another factor. The hypothesis regarding potential effect modifiers should be formulated prior to data collection and analysis, based on the previous evidence. It can be evaluated by subdividing the data into strata of the potential effect modifier and by assessing the effect of the trigger on the outcome across the levels of the effect modifier. For example, in the study of the effect of anger on the risk of myocardial infarction (the Onset Study), the investigators considered effect modification by use of aspirin (4). After stratifying by aspirin use they found that the estimated relative risk of myocardial infarction associated with anger was lower among regular users of aspirin than among nonusers (4).

One can also test statistically for difference in odds ratios across the strata by applying the chi-squared test of homogeneity. For further discussion on statistical tests of homogeneity of odds ratios, see Rothman and Greenland (15).

5.3 NESTED CASE-COHORT DESIGN

Large cohort studies contain features that affect their efficiency and validity:

1. One is usually able to obtain limited data on almost everyone in the cohort, some of which may be subject to errors of measurement.
2. One may be able to collect or obtain more data on the study subjects using more intensive resources. Such data may include information obtained from biological measurements, intensive review of records, or interviewing.
3. One may need or be able to study a smaller number of subjects without loss of validity by using nested designs.

This section will discuss the main features of nested designs that pertain to the case-control method. In particular, we will cover methods for selecting cases and controls within a cohort study, as well as the main principles of analysis of the case-cohort design. The nested designs discussed below, however, are more closely related to the cohort method and for that reason will not be discussed in great detail.

Case-based designs can be conducted within a larger cohort and they are called "nested." Nested case-based designs utilize information on exposure and other covariates on all individuals who develop the outcome (cases), as well as on individuals in the comparison group, rather than all members of the cohort. These designs, therefore, improve efficiency of the cohort study by reducing the amount of information and other resources needed to address the research question.

Nested designs possess the key features of case-based designs as well as some methodological advantages. As with any other case-based designs, these are based on a comparative approach of persons with a certain outcome with persons who do not have the outcome. Nested designs are also advantageous in establishing antecedence of exposure, since the relevant exposure information is usually collected prior to the information on the outcome becomes available. Finally, nested designs also enjoy the advantages of the cohort design as they allow for studying changes in exposure that occur over time.

There are two major groups of nested designs—nested case-control and nested case-cohort designs—and which one is used depends on how the comparison group is selected. The key feature of a nested case-control design is that all cases and nondiseased comparison subjects or controls are selected from the same base population or from the same cohort. As all case-control studies can eventually identify such a base population, there are those who assume that all case-control studies are nested. The most common version of a nested case-control design is when controls are selected at the same time that the case develops among cohort members who were at risk of becoming cases at the same point in time. These potential controls are the individuals within the cohort who did not develop the disease at earlier times and those who were not lost to follow-up at the moment when the case developed. This type of sampling is called *incidence density sampling*.

The mechanism of selecting the comparison group in a case-cohort study is quite different. In a case-cohort study the comparison group, called a *sub-cohort*, is selected at random from the initial cohort at baseline regardless of the outcome. The sub-cohort becomes the comparison group for all cases. Therefore, investigators need to compile information on exposure and other characteristics of all cases and the members of the sub-cohort, which improves the study efficiency. No other member of the overall cohort is included in the analysis. However, since the sub-cohort is selected at the initiation of the overall cohort, some members of the sub-cohort may develop the disease or be lost to follow-up (see Figure 5.3). The composition of the sub-cohort is, therefore, dynamic. Individuals in the sub-cohort who develop the outcome of interest are excluded from the comparison group once they become a "case."

Gunter et al. conducted a case-cohort study of hyperinsulinemia and the risk of colorectal cancer nested within the Women's Health

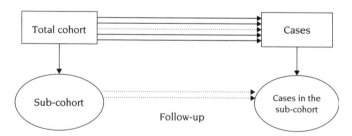

Figure 5.3. Schematic Representation of the Nested Case-Cohort Design

Note: One-sided arrows represent the study participants who develop the outcome and become cases during the follow-up: both outside (upper part of the diagram) and inside (lower part of the diagram) the sub-cohort.

Initiative Observational Study (16). The investigators analyzed serum specimens of 438 women who developed colorectal cancer as well as of 816 women in the sub-cohort selected at random from all women of the initial cohort. As the original cohort consisted of 93,676 women, the decision to conduct a nested case-cohort study led to a significant gain in resources.

Analysis of case-cohort data involves use of the Cox proportional hazards model with correction for correlation related to the design (17). Construction of the model includes careful consideration for when the risk for development of the outcome stops and starts for each study participant. These times are different for members of the sub-cohort than for the cases outside of the sub-cohort. For the members of the sub-cohort the time of the beginning of risk is the time of cohort initiation, while the end is either the end of the follow-up or the time when they develop the disease. The cases outside of the sub-cohort are not considered at risk for developing the outcome until the time just prior to becoming a case. Their end time is the time when they become a case (17).

5.4 HIGHLIGHTS OF THE CASE-COHORT DESIGN

1. In a case-cohort study, no assumption is made that the comparison group consists of noncases, and as some cases of the disease may be part of the comparison group, this method can be used to study some common conditions with a large number of subclinical cases such as arthritis.
2. As a result of point 1 it is not necessary to abide by the rare disease assumption when designing and analyzing a case-cohort study.
3. The random sub-cohort selected as the comparison group will allow for the estimation of the frequency of exposure variables in the base population.
4. The study may be able to use one sub-cohort comparison group to assess relationships with more than one outcome of interest by comparing more than one case group to the members of the sub-cohort.

REFERENCES

1. Hosoglu S, Aldemir M, Akalin S, Geyik MF, Tacyldiz IH, Loeb M. Risk factors for enteric perforation in patients with typhoid fever. *Am J Epidemiol.* 2004;160:46-50.
2. Maclure M. The case-crossover design: a method for studying transient effects on the risk of acute events. *Am J Epidemiol.* 1991;133:144-153.

3. Armenian HK. Genetic and environmental factors in the aetiology of familial paroxysmal polyserositis. An analysis of 150 cases from Lebanon. *Trop Geogr Med.* 1982;34(2):183-187.

4. Mittleman MA, Maclure M, Sherwood JB, et al. Triggering of acute myocardial infarction onset by episodes of anger. Determinants of Myocardial Infarction Onset Study Investigators. *Circulation.* 1995;92(7):1720-1725.

5. Mittleman MA, Maclure M, Tofler GH, Sherwood JB, Goldberg RJ, Muller JE. Triggering of acute myocardial infarction by heavy physical exertion. Protection against triggering by regular exertion. Determinants of Myocardial Infarction Onset Study Investigators. *N Engl J Med.* 1993;329(23):1677-1683.

6. Hernandez-Diaz S, Hernan MA, Meyer K, Werler MM, Mitchell AA. Case-crossover and case-time-control designs in birth defects epidemiology. *Am J Epidemiol.* 2003;158(4):385-391.

7. Sorock GS, Lombardi DA, Hauser R, Eisen EA, Herrick RF, Mittleman MA. A case-crossover study of transient risk factors for occupational acute hand injury. *Occup Environ Med.* 2004;61(4):305-311.

8. Polevoi SK, Quinn JV, Kramer NR. Factors associated with patients who leave without being seen. *Acad Emerg Med.* 2005;12(3):232-236.

9. Symons JM, Wang L, Guallar E, et al. A case-crossover study of fine particulate matter air pollution and onset of congestive heart failure symptom exacerbation leading to hospitalization. *Am J Epidemiol.* 2006;164(5):421-433.

10. Schneider MF, Gange SJ, Margolick JB, et al. Application of case-crossover and case-time-control study designs in analyses of time-varying predictors of T-cell homeostasis failure. *Ann Epidemiol.* 2005;55: 137-144.

11. Armenian HK, Lilienfeld AM. Incubation period of disease. *Epidemiologic Reviews.* 1983;5:1-15.

12. Navidi W. Bidirectional case-crossover designs for exposures with time trends. *Biometrics.* 1998;54(2):596-605.

13. Breslow NE, Day NE. Classical methods of analysis of matched data. *Statistical Methods in Cancer Research, Volume I, The Analysis of Case-Control Studies,* chapter 5:. Lyon: IARC Scientific Publications; 1980:162-189.

14. Breslow NE, Day NE. Conditional logistic regression for matched sets. *Statistical Methods in Cancer Research, Volume I, The Analysis of Case-Control Studies,* chapter 7. Lyon: IARC Scientific Publications; 1980:246-279.

15. Rothman KJ, Greenland S. Introduction to stratified analysis. *Modern Epidemiology,* chapter 15. Lippincott – Raven; 1998:253-279.

16. Gunter MJ, Hoover DR, Yu H, et al. Insulin, insulin-like growth factor-I, endogenous estradiol, and risk of colorectal cancer in postmenopausal women. *Cancer Res.* 2008;68 (1): 329-337.

17. Barlow WE, Ichikawa L, Rosner D, Izumi S. Analysis of case-cohort designs. *J Clin Epidemiol.* 1999;52(12):1165-1172.

6

ANALYSIS OF CASE-CONTROL DATA

Gayane Yenokyan

OUTLINE

This chapter aims to

1. present the main steps in the analysis of case-control data;
2. discuss some of the challenges related to the analysis of case-control data;
3. list common strategies of dealing with confounding and effect modification in the analysis; and
4. discuss interpretation and presentation of the results of the analysis.

6.1 INTRODUCTION TO ANALYSIS

This chapter will cover the analysis of unmatched case-control data, as well as matched data as a special case. The main steps in the analysis presented below are relevant to the analysis of *any* data. They will then be discussed in further detail. Along with discussing the overall strategy, the peculiarities related to case-control data analysis will be emphasized. The main steps are

1. formulating and focusing on the study hypothesis;
2. exploring the data;
3. carrying out bivariate analysis;
4. carrying out multivariate analysis;
5. presenting and interpreting the results.

6.1.1 Study Hypothesis

The study hypothesis is usually formulated at the early stages of the epidemiological investigation. The relationship between study hypothesis and data analysis is bidirectional. On one hand, proper formulation of study hypothesis defines the boundaries of data acquisition and analysis. On the other hand, it is successful data analysis that properly incorporates and addresses the study hypothesis. Therefore, the study hypothesis should have all the necessary elements for drawing inferences about the relationship between the exposure and the outcome of interest.

The essential elements of the study hypothesis include *definition of outcome and exposure of interest, the direction of the relationship between the outcome and the exposure,* as well as the *specific population relevant to the relationship.* For example, in a study of the effect of patient education on adherence to prescribed medication, one of the study hypotheses can be formulated as "knowledge of cardiovascular risk factors increases the proportion of patients who take the prescribed medications a year after prior cardio-vascular event." This definition includes *measurable* exposure, knowledge of cardiovascular risk factors, the *outcome*, taking medications after a year since they were prescribed, *the specific population* the hypothesis is applicable to, patients with prior cardiovascular events, as well as defines the possible direction of the relationship between the exposure and the outcome.

The proper formulation of the study hypothesis is critical for causal inferences between the exposure and the outcome. To make a causal statement about the studied relationship, it is essential to be able to assume that no other factor that might affect the estimated relationship between the exposure and the outcome, that is, confounder, is left out of the analysis. Further, to be able to incorporate these factors in the analysis, the researcher must fully understand (to the extent possible) how the exposure affects the outcome and what these other relevant factors are. For an extended discussion of how study design and background knowledge on the relationship between exposure and outcome play an important role in defining the boundaries of data analysis, see Robins (1). These considerations should be made at the planning stage of a study by collecting data on the relevant factors.

Another important consideration for data analysis is how closely the exposure, outcome, and all relevant factors are measured. Potential bias in exposure measurement is covered in Chapter 4.

6.1.2 *Exploratory Data Analysis*

Exploratory data analysis is perhaps the most important aspect of any data analysis, and is often overlooked. According to Diggle, Liang, and Zeger, "Exploratory data analysis is detective work. It comprises techniques to visualize patterns in data" (2). Looking at the data at hand aims to

1. reveal unusual and outlying observations;
2. assess the amount of missing data on exposure, outcome, and other relevant variables;
3. discover systematic relationships that are relevant to the study hypothesis.

6.1.2.1 *Editing and cleaning data.* The first step in the exploratory data analysis includes *editing and cleaning* the data for possible data errors. The analyst should always make sure that values of all variables in the dataset are legitimate by studying the ranges and the distributions of the variables. Graphical displays as well as simple summaries of data are usually helpful in identifying possible errors.

6.1.2.2 *Assessing missing data.* Before embarking on the analysis of the data, the analyst needs to assess the *amount and the distribution of the missing data*. The reasons for missing data should also be explored. For example, the number of cigarettes smoked last year is expected to be missing among nonsmokers, while among smokers the reason for missing data on cigarettes needs to be investigated. Depending on the amount and the mechanism of missing data, there are different approaches to dealing with this problem. The methods range from limiting the data analysis to the "complete cases," that is, persons with nonmissing values on all the variables of interest, and leaving out the missing observations, to imputing the missing data based on the values of other covariates.

For a conceptual discussion see Rubin (3), and for its application in data analysis see Harrell (4).

Once possible errors have been corrected, the analysis should proceed toward exploring meaningful relationships in the data that are relevant to addressing the study hypothesis. For example, in a study of the effect of patient knowledge on adherence to medication, the adherence to medication can be plotted against the knowledge score. One useful technique is to use the *lowess*—locally weighted regression scatter plot smoothing—method (5). This method plots the local average of the response variable (outcome) against the predictor (exposure) and allows visualizing the relationship between the response and the predictor. Since in case-control studies the outcome is binary, it is possible to plot a logit-transformed lowess curve; for example, the log odds of being adherent to medication would be plotted against the knowledge score. This technique is extremely useful for exploring nonlinear relationships between the response and the predictor variable. Major inflection points on the graph should be considered as evidence for modeling a nonlinear relationship, for example, using linear splines.

Similar graphs can be used to investigate the relationship between the outcome and potential confounders. The knowledge of this relationship will allow for better representation of the confounders in the model and ultimately will lead to better adjustment. We will discuss confounding and model-building strategies in later sections of this chapter.

6.1.2.3 Selecting continuous predictors. Relevant to exploring the relationship between variables is *selection of the functional form of continuous predictors.* The main options here are to

1. categorize continuous predictors based on some criteria;
2. include continuous variables as they are;
3. model nonlinear relationships by including linear or cubic splines or fractional polynomials.

Categorization of continuous predictors is fairly common in epidemiological studies. Advantages of this approach include use of stratified analysis, ease of interpretation, and in some cases more direct application to clinical or public health practice. For example, in a study of plasma urate levels and risk of Parkinson's disease, the investigators opted to categorize the exposure into quartiles, which were defined according to the distribution of plasma urate in the controls (6). Other continuous variables were categorized as well: alcohol use was split into categories based on use per day (0, 1–9, 10–19, 20–29, 30 and above grams per day), regular aspirin use was dichotomized (greater than 2 per week or less), and categories of other variables were defined based on their distributions in controls (6).

The following criteria are often used to categorize continuous variables (7):

- Biologically relevant ranges, to represent separate categories—for example, female age before, during, and after childbearing age or menopause;
- Clinically defined cutoffs—for example, accepted normal values, below normal, and above normal;
- Categories used in other studies to enable comparisons across different studies—for example, many studies classify body mass index (BMI) into underweight (<18.5), normal (18.5–25), overweight (25–30), and obese (>30) categories;
- Categories based on the distribution of continuous variables (usually quartiles or quintiles);
- Categories based on natural cutoffs of the distribution, as in a clearly bimodal or tri-modal distribution.

More recent research into categorization of continuous variables revealed that statistically categorization of continuous variables might lead to loss of information, false positive associations, and reduced power to reveal the true associations (7). Further, categorization of confounding variables might lead to only partial adjustment and residual confounding. In spite of these developments, categorization still remains an attractive option in presenting and interpreting results of case-control studies.

Depending on the results of the exploratory analysis, any of the above mentioned approaches might work as long as they do not contradict the natural relationship between the outcome and the continuous variable in the data. For example, the relationship might appear linear (Figure 6.1). In this case the variable can be included in the model by itself. In other cases the relationship might appear as in Figure 6.2.

Here homogenous groups can be represented by a single risk category and categorization can be considered.

One can also test for nonlinear relationships by including linear splines or higher-order predictors, such as quadratic or cubic terms in the model. The analyst can test whether the coefficient for the quadratic term is significantly different from zero. If the null hypothesis can be rejected at a predetermined level of statistical significance (in most cases, 0.05), one can reasonably conclude that the relationship between

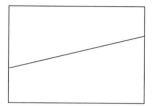

Figure 6.1. Linear Relationship of Continuous Variable and Outcome

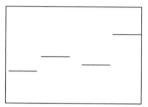

Figure 6.2. Categorical Relationship of Continuous Variable and Outcome

the outcome and the predictor of interest is not linear, but quadratic. For further discussion see Harrell (8).

6.1.2.4 *Stratified analysis.* One of the main advantages of the use of categories for both exposure variables and confounders is the ability to carry out stratified analysis. In stratified analysis the investigator divides the data into groups (strata) specified by the value of a third variable to look at the relationship between the exposure and the outcome. For example, in a study of patient knowledge of cardiovascular risk factors and adherence to prescribed medications one could stratify by patients' sex to look at the relationship between the exposure and the outcome within people of the same sex. What the stratified analysis achieves is to remove the effect of the stratified variable, that is, sex, from the relationship between the exposure and the outcome.

Stratified analysis can be useful in

- adjusting for known and measured confounders;
- checking for heterogeneity of the measure of association across the groups (strata) (9);
- performing subgroup analysis.

As outlined in Chapter 4, the odds ratio approximates relative risk in measuring the association between exposure and outcome in case-control studies. The odds ratio might be confounded by the presence of other factors that are predictive of the outcome. In order to affect the odds ratio, the factors need to be differentially distributed among the exposed and the unexposed in the study population. In modern epidemiology the following three criteria are used to define confounding:

1. The confounder causally affects the outcome.
2. The confounder is distributed differentially among the exposed and the unexposed in the study population in the data.
3. The confounder is not affected by the exposure.

For example, on the left-hand side in Figure 6.3, the confounder affects the outcome and the exposure, and is not affected by the exposure. On the right-hand side, however, since the factor is affected by exposure, it does not confound the relationship between the exposure and the outcome. More on the use of diagrams in confounder diagnostics and some useful examples can be found in Merchant and Pitiphat (10).

One of the earliest methods of control for known and measured confounders is stratified analysis. (The reason we emphasize that the confounder should be known and measured is that it is impossible to consider confounding by unknown factors as well as factors for which the study has not collected any data.) As previously discussed, by creating groups, or strata, with the same value of the confounder (in our example, sex), the investigator eliminates the effect of the confounder within each strata.

An additional supporting criterion for confounding diagnostics is that in the presence of confounding the observed crude odds ratio is considerably different from the stratum-specific odds ratios. The next section will discuss the Mantel-Haenszel odds ratio as the method to pull information from stratum-specific odds ratios into a single adjusted measure.

6.1.2.5. *Mantel-Haenszel estimates.* The initial step of data analysis is usually to estimate the ratio of odds of exposure among cases and controls, or the odds ratio. This estimate is called crude odds ratio. In observational research, crude odds ratio is usually confounded by the factors that affect the risk of developing the outcome or confounders. Therefore, the next step is to remove the effect of the confounder and to determine if this will result in a change of odds ratio.

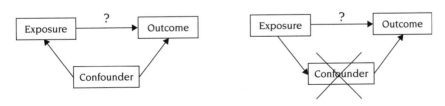

Figure 6.3. Confounder, Exposure, and Outcome Relationships

In the presence of confounding, the stratum-specific odds ratios (odds ratios in each stratum of the confounding variable) are usually different from the crude odds ratio. Further, the odds ratios across strata are numerically very close. The diagram below summarizes the behavior of crude, stratified, and stratum-specific odds ratios in the presence of confounding.

$$OR_{crude} \neq OR_{stratified}$$

$$OR_{stratum1} \cong OR_{stratum2} \cong \ldots \cong OR_{stratum\ K}$$

Assuming the factor by which the data were stratified is the only confounder (a rather unreasonable assumption in most epidemiological studies), the stratified odds ratio represents the true relationship between the exposure and the outcome. The next paragraph discusses how the stratified odds ratio is calculated.

The stratified odds ratio is a measure that combines the stratum-specific odds ratios that are homogenous with respect to the confounding variable and therefore are free of its influence. The Mantel-Haenszel method combines stratum-specific odds ratios (or any other measures of association) into one combined estimate, the Mantel-Haenszel odds ratio.

This method was proposed by Mantel and Haenszel in their 1959 paper "Statistical Aspects of the Analysis of Data from Retrospective Studies of Disease" (11). According to this method, the Mantel-Haenszel estimator is equal to,

$$OR_{MH} = \frac{\sum_i \dfrac{A_i \times D_i}{N_i}}{\sum_i \dfrac{B_i \times C_i}{N_i}},$$

where cells A, D, B, C are specified as in Figure 6.4, and index i represents each stratum.

Consider the following two strata of a confounder C in looking at the relationship between a disease, D and an exposure, E: if there are only two strata, the

$$OR_{MH} = \frac{\dfrac{A_1 \times D_1}{N_1} + \dfrac{A_0 \times D_0}{N_0}}{\dfrac{B_1 \times C_1}{N_1} + \dfrac{B_0 \times C_0}{N_0}}$$

		D=1	D=1	
C=1	E=1	A1	B1	
	E=0	C1	D1	
				N1

		D=1	D=0	
C=0	E=1	A0	B0	
	E=0	C0	D0	
				N0

Figure 6.4. Relationship of Outcome D and Exposure E in Two Strata of a Confounder C

The calculated Mantel-Haenszel odds ratio is now adjusted for the confounder C. The Mantel-Haenszel stratified odds ratio can be calculated for a limited number of categorical covariates. If, however, the main exposure or some of the confounders are continuous, it is more efficient to use multivariate adjustment techniques.

6.1.2.6 *Multivariate analysis.* Multivariate analysis allows estimating the relationship between exposure and outcome, having removed the effect of potential confounders. Since in case-control studies the outcome is binary (presence or absence of a disease or other condition), the most common regression used for analysis of case-control data is logistic regression.

From Chapter 4 we know that the odds of any event are defined as the ratio of probability of experiencing the event and the probability of not having the event.

$$odds = \frac{\Pr(event)}{1 - \Pr(event)}$$

Logistic regression models natural logarithm of odds of outcome as a function of the exposure and other covariates,

$$\log(odds) = \beta_0 + \beta_1 Z + \sum_{i=2}^{p} \beta_i X_i, \qquad (1)$$

where Z is the exposure of interest, and X_i are other covariates in the model.

Given the model, β_1 is interpreted as the difference in log odds of outcome comparing exposed to unexposed at a fixed level of other covariates. Again, as in stratified analysis we compare exposed to unexposed among patients who possess the same value of potential confounders (here, X_is), so that these confounders do not influence the estimated relationship between exposure and outcome.

To obtain the estimated odds ratio, the estimate of difference in log odds, β_1 needs to be exponentiated. The sign of the beta estimate indicates the direction of the relationship between the exposure and the outcome (see Table 6.1).

The standard regression output usually includes standard errors as well as confidence intervals for the beta coefficients at any required level of statistical significance. Based on this information the analyst can test a hypothesis about the beta coefficient. The most common hypothesis to test would be whether the data provide enough evidence to discard a possibility of no relationship between the exposure and the outcome. This is equivalent to testing whether $\beta_1 = 0$ under the null hypothesis. If the observed data and the test statistic are considerably large, one can conclude that data are far from being compatible with the null hypothesis of no relationship between the exposure and the outcome. The conclusion in this case would be that there is in fact a relationship, either positive or negative, between the exposure and the outcome.

Let us consider the following example of a case-control study of analgesic drug use and risk of ovarian cancer (12). This study included 812 women aged 25 to 74 diagnosed with ovarian cancer and 1,313 controls. Use of analgesics was the main exposure variable. The authors looked at different kinds of drugs (acetaminophen, aspirin, and others) and duration of use, as well as indication for use. Logistic regression was used to estimate the effect of analgesics on developing ovarian cancer.

The authors used logistic regression to estimate the odds ratio of ovarian cancer and a 95% confidence interval. The authors adjusted for potential confounders, factors related to the outcome, such as age, country of residence, year of diagnosis, number of full-term pregnancies, and duration of hormonal contraception. Additional confounders were also considered (12).

The investigators found a positive, statistically significant relationship between analgesic drug use and the development of ovarian cancer. The

Table 6.1. Beta Estimates and the Relationship between the Exposure and the Outcome

$\beta_1 = 0$	No relationship between the exposure and the outcome: exposed and unexposed have the same odds of outcome
$\beta_1 > 0$	Positive relationship between the exposure and the outcome: exposed patients have *higher* odds of outcome compared to the unexposed
$\beta_1 < 0$	Negative relationship between the exposure and the outcome: exposed patients have *lower* odds of outcome compared to the unexposed

adjusted odds ratio of ovarian cancer comparing ever users of nonsteroidal anti-inflammatory drugs to never users was 1.2 with a 95% confidence interval 1.0, 1.4. This result can be interpreted in the following manner: comparing women of the same age, country of residence, year of diagnosis, number of full-term pregnancies, and duration of hormonal contraception, those who ever used nonsteroidal anti-inflammatory drugs are at 20% higher risk of ovarian cancer than nonusers.

6.1.2.7 *Testing for interaction.* The relationship between the exposure and the outcome might be different depending on the level of a third variable. In this case the third variable is called the effect modifier, and the phenomenon is effect modification. If effect modification is present, it must be reflected in the analysis.

First, how does the researcher identify that effect modification is present? In some cases the effect modification has been described in previous studies. For example, smoking worsens the negative impact of oral contraceptives on cardiovascular mortality. In this case smoking is the effect modifier, since it "modifies" the effect of oral contraceptives on cardiovascular disease.

In other cases effect modification can be hypothesized based on the available information about the mechanism of the relationship between exposure and outcome. This needs to be done at the planning stage of case-control study, so that information on the potential effect modifier is collected. At the analysis stage, the analyst can statistically test for effect modification by including an interaction term in the model and testing for its significance.

A model with interaction might appear as below:

$$\log(odds) = \beta_0 + \beta_1 Z + \beta_2 V + \beta_3 (Z \times V) + \sum_{i=4}^{p} \beta_i X_i, \qquad (2)$$

where Z is the exposure of interest and V is the potential effect modifier. The product of Z and V is called interaction term.

If the interaction term is included in the model, it means that the model assumes that the relationship between Z and the outcome is different depending on whether V is present or absent (This simplest case can be easily generalized to V having more than two categories, or when V is continuous).

To illustrate effect modification mathematically, we can rearrange the terms in the above model as follows:

$$\log(odds) = \beta_0 + (\beta_1 + \beta_3 V) Z + \beta_2 V + \sum_{i=4}^{p} \beta_i X_i. \qquad (3)$$

We can see that the beta coefficient for Z, the exposure, is now not just β_1 as before, but is $\beta_1 + \beta_3 V$, and therefore depends on the value of V. In the simplest case, when V can either be 0 or 1 (absent or present, smoker or nonsmoker), the estimated effect of exposure will be β_1 if V is 0; it will be $\beta_1 + \beta_3$ if V is 1. We can see, therefore, that the effect of exposure changes depending on the presence or absence of V, and this difference is β_3. If, however, β_3 is 0, we will go back to the model (eqn 1) without interaction:

$$\log(odds) = \beta_0 + \beta_1 Z + \sum_{i=2}^{p} \beta_i X_i$$

This means that when the analyst suspects that a certain factor might act as an effect modifier, he or she can include an interaction term in a model and test whether the data provide enough evidence to reject the null hypothesis that the coefficient on the interaction term is equal to zero, $\beta_3 = 0$. Depending on the results of the test, the model that is more adequate for the data at hand could be the one with (eqn 2) or without (eqn 1) interaction.

To illustrate the effect modification in an epidemiological study, let us consider the following example. A study was conducted to determine if the effect of oral contraceptive use on ovarian cancer differs by menopausal status (13). Based on earlier data and reported associations in pre- and postmenopausal women, the authors hypothesized that menopausal status might act as an effect modifier in the relationship between oral contraceptive use and risk of ovarian cancer. Specifically, they assumed that the association between the exposure and the outcome is stronger in premenopausal than in postmenopausal women.

To assess the presence of effect modification by menopausal status, the authors included a product (i.e., interaction) term for menopausal status and oral contraceptive use in the models (13, p. 1061). As we have learned, statistically, effect modification is evaluated by the test of significance of the interaction term. The test indicates whether sufficient evidence exists in the data to reject the null hypothesis of absence of effect modification. If the null hypothesis is rejected, one can conclude that the interaction (effect modification) is significant. In the study of oral contraceptive use and ovarian cancer, the authors found that the interaction term was significant for the main exposure and for the duration of use (p-values = 0.022 and 0.03, respectively).

Let us further consider the actual models for estimating the effect of oral contraceptive use in pre- and postmenopausal women. The odds ratios and the 95% confidence intervals are presented in table 3

(13, p.1063). The odds ratio for oral contraceptive use (adjusted for age, race, family history of cancer, age at menarche, tubal ligation, infertility, body mass index, number of full-term pregnancies, and age at last pregnancy) was 0.5 (95% confidence interval: 0.3, 0.8) among premenopausal women, and 0.8 (95% confidence interval: 0.6, 1.1) among postmenopausal women. How were these estimates obtained?

One can obtain the estimated odds ratios for oral contraceptive use in pre- and postmenopausal women by running a model with interaction term.

The model with interaction can be rewritten as

$$\log(\text{odds of cancer}) = \beta_0 + \beta_1 OC + \beta_2 \text{ postmenopausal}$$
$$+ \beta_3 OC \times \text{postmenopausal} + \sum_4^p \beta_p X_p,$$

where OC stands for oral contraceptive use.

It is important to note the variable coding in this model: OC users are coded "1" and nonusers are coded "0." Postmenopausal women are coded as "1" and premenopausal women are coded as "0."

To make the interpretation of coefficients a little easier, we should further rewrite the model above as model (eqn 3) above:

$$\log(\text{odds of cancer}) = \beta_0 + \beta_2 \text{ postmenopausal}$$
$$+ (\beta_1 + \beta_3 \text{ postmenopausal}) OC + \sum_4^p \beta_p X_p.$$

We need the estimates of the effect of oral contraceptives in two groups of women. For premenopausal women, the variable *postmenopausal* will be "0," and the model will be reduced to

$$\log(\text{odds of cancer}) = \beta_0 + \beta_1 OC + \beta_2 \text{ postmenopausal} + \sum_4^p \beta_p X_p$$

The coefficient on OC, β_1, estimates the log odds ratio of cancer comparing OC users and nonusers among premenopausal women and adjusted for all other covariates in the model. To obtain the reported estimate of 0.5, one should exponentiate β_1.

For postmenopausal women, the variable *postmenopausal* will be "1," and the resulting model will be:

$$\log(\text{odds of cancer}) = \beta_0 + \beta_2 \text{ postmenopausal} + (\beta_1 + \beta_3) OC + \sum_4^p \beta_p X_p$$

The estimate of log odds ratio of cancer comparing OC users to nonusers in postmenopausal women will then be $\beta_1 + \beta_3$. After exponentiating the sum $\beta_1 + \beta_3$, the analyst will have the odds ratio of cancer comparing OC users to nonusers in postmenopausal women and adjusted for all other covariates in the model. This value, according to the authors, was 0.8.

Here we demonstrated how the epidemiological research question about effect modification can be addressed using the statistical tools.

6.1.3 Analysis of Matched Data

As discussed in Chapter 3, the purpose of matching is to achieve comparability of cases and controls by creating groups with roughly similar distributions of the potential confounders, or the matching factors. The chapter also outlined different types of matching (individual vs. frequency) as well as advantages and disadvantages of matching. This section will describe how the analysis of matched data differs from the analysis of unmatched case-control studies.

The initial steps of analysis of matched data do not differ from those for the analysis of unmatched data. The analyst should still proceed through formulating and focusing on the study hypothesis and conducting exploratory analysis of the data.

The bivariate and multivariate analyses are different and should account for the matched data.

The simplest case of matching is one-to-one individually matched data. In one-to-one matched data, cases and controls are grouped in pairs and have the same value of the matching variable(s). The pairs represent matched "sets," within which the value of the exposure variable could be either the same ("concordant" sets) or different ("discordant" sets).

For example, Table 6.2 presents hypothetical data, where the sets (pairs) 1, 4, 7, 9, and 10 are concordant, and the sets 2, 3, 5, 6, and 8 are discordant with regard to exposure.

6.1.3.1 *Bivariate analysis of matched data.* In the analysis of matched case-control data, only the sets that are discordant with regard to exposure contribute to the analysis.

To understand why this is the case, one should remember the purpose of the analysis of case-control data. The goal of designing and implementing case-control studies is to evaluate whether exposure is associated with outcome, or, in other words, whether the cases are more likely to be exposed than the controls (positive association between exposure and the outcome) or whether the cases are less likely to be exposed than the controls (negative association). With matching, the data come in

Table 6.2. Hypothetical Matched
Case-Control Data

Pair	Case	Control
1	exposed	exposed
2	exposed	unexposed
3	unexposed	exposed
4	unexposed	unexposed
5	exposed	unexposed
6	exposed	unexposed
7	exposed	exposed
8	unexposed	exposed
9	unexposed	unexposed
10	unexposed	unexposed

sets. If both the case and the control within the matched set are exposed or unexposed, this information is not helpful in answering the question of whether cases are more or less likely to be exposed than controls. Therefore, the concordant sets are noninformative regarding the association between exposure and the outcome, and the analysis mainly focuses on discordant sets.

Next, the analysis has to distinguish between the discordant sets in which the case is exposed (and the control is unexposed), and the sets in which the control is exposed (and the case is unexposed). These two types of sets both answer the question of association, but they contribute to different directions of the association. If more sets contain exposed cases than unexposed cases, the association between the exposure and the outcome is probably positive. In this case, those who have the outcome (i.e., cases) are more exposed than those who do not have the outcome (i.e., controls). The opposite is true as well: if there are more discordant sets with exposed controls, the association between the outcome and the exposure is likely to be negative. In this case, absence (not the presence) of the outcome, that is, being a control, is related to having the exposure, so the association between outcome and exposure is negative or protective.

With these considerations in mind, it is natural to subclassify the discordant sets into sets with exposed cases and sets with exposed controls. The simplest method to do this is by using a 2 × 2 table. (Note that this 2 × 2 table differs from the one described earlier in this chapter and that the numbers in the cells represent pairs of cases and controls rather than individuals.)

Using the hypothetical example of 10 matched pairs above, we have Table 6.3.

The odds ratio in a one-to-one matched case-control study is estimated as a ratio of the two types of discordant pairs: the number of

Table 6.3. Summary Data of Table 6.2

		Control	
		Exposed	Unexposed
Case	Exposed	2	3
	Unexposed	2	3

Table 6.4. Tabular Presentation for Matched Data Analysis

		Control	
		Exposed	Unexposed
Case	Exposed	a	b
	Unexposed	c	d

pairs in which the case is exposed to the number of pairs in which the control is exposed.

Based on Table 6.3, the estimate of the odds ratio is $3/2 = 1.5$

In general, given Table 6.4, the estimate of the matched odds ratio is b/c.

Given the result, the analyst can also test the null hypothesis of no association between exposure and outcome. This is equivalent to testing whether the true odds ratio is "1," or whether the numbers of discordant pairs are equal, $b = c$. The test is called McNemar's test and the estimate is the McNemar's odds ratio (14).

To calculate the confidence interval around the estimated odds ratio, we can use the formula for the standard error (SE) of the natural logarithm of the odds ratio (OR):

$$SE(\log OR) = \sqrt{\frac{1}{b} + \frac{1}{c}}$$

where b is the number of pairs with an exposed case, and c is the number of pairs with an exposed control.

In our example, the estimate of the standard error will be:

$$SE(\log OR) = \sqrt{\frac{1}{3} + \frac{1}{2}} = 0.91$$

In order to use the standard error to calculate a $(100 - \alpha)$ confidence interval for the true odds ratio, we need the logarithm of the estimated odds ratio. Using that value, we will first calculate a confidence interval for the logarithm of the odds ratio. This interval can be translated into a confidence interval for the odds ratio by exponentiating its lower and upper bounds. To illustrate this process, let us compute the 95% confidence interval for the odds ratio in our hypothetical example above.

First, we need the natural logarithm of the estimated odds ratio:

$$\log(OR) = \log(1.5) = 0.405$$

The upper and the lower bounds of the 95% confidence interval are calculated using the formula below:

$$\log(OR) \pm SE(\log OR) \times Z_{\alpha/2}$$

where $Z_{\alpha/2}$ is the value of the standard normal variate corresponding to $\alpha/2$ area under the curve. For the 95% confidence interval is equal $Z_{\alpha/2}$ to 1.96.

Therefore, the upper and the lower bounds of the 95% confidence interval for the logarithm of odds ratio in our example will be:

$$\log(OR) \pm SE(\log OR) \times Z_{\alpha/2} = 0.405 \pm 0.91 \times 1.96 = -1.38, 2.19$$

Lastly, this interval needs to be converted into a confidence interval for the odds ratio. For this we exponentiate the numbers above and we calculate:

95% confidence interval for OR = exp(−1.38), exp(2.19)
$$= 0.25, 8.94.$$

6.1.3.2 *Multivariate analysis of matched data—Conditional logistic regression.* The bivariate analysis presented in the previous section only allows us to look at the relationship between a dichotomous exposure or other covariate and the outcome. To be able to assess relationships between continuous exposures and the outcome, as well as to look at adjusted relationships, the analyst should use bivariate or multivariate modeling techniques. The standard method for modeling individually matched data is a conditional logistic regression analysis.

Conditional logistic regression provides estimates of log conditional odds ratios for the variables included in the model. However, it can only estimate the log odds ratio for the variables, which differ between cases and controls. Thus, the log odds ratio cannot be estimated for a variable for which cases and controls have the same value or match exactly. For example, if cases and controls are matched on gender, then within the matched sets all of the cases and controls are either males or females, that is, they have the same value of the matching variable. In this situation, the odds ratio for gender cannot be estimated.

One can, however, look at effect modification by the matching factors using conditional logistic regression. If in the above example of matching on gender, the main exposure is aspirin use and the investigators suspect that the effect of aspirin use on the outcome might be different in men and women, they can create an interaction term and test for its significance using conditional logistic regression. In this case the interaction term will include a product of aspirin use (the main exposure) and gender (the matching factor). Test of the significance of the interaction term will provide evidence for the differential effect of aspirin on the outcome in men and women (effect modification).

Some statistical software programs, such as STATA, allow direct estimation of coefficients using conditional logistic regression. Others, such as SAS, need some extra programming to accommodate fitting conditional logistic regression. This can be done by employing conditional likelihood methods used for the Cox proportional hazards model (15).

A simpler extension of standard logistic regression technique is available for use for one-to-one matched data. First, the unit of analysis needs to be the matched set, which reduces the total sample size to the number of case-control pairs. Second, to estimate the value of the coefficients the analyst needs to define a new variable to represent the difference between the case and the control within each matched pair. This variable is then used in the standard logistic regression as the covariate for which the coefficient will be estimated. Finally, one needs to use standard logistic regression with no intercept. More on how logistic regression can be used to fit matched data, including extension to one-to-M matched designs can be found in Hosmer and Lemeshow (2000), (15, pp. 226-252).

6.2 MODEL BUILDING

One of the most common questions that an analyst faces is the formulation of the model. However, if the study hypothesis is appropriately defined, one can estimate the relationships of interest effectively using statistical tools. For example, once the exposure of interest is carefully defined and measured, it can easily be included in the model to assess its relationship with the outcome. Next, if appropriate confounding diagnostics are carried out, especially prior to any data collection, the scope of potential covariates in the model will be also well defined. Finally, any potential effect modifiers should also be considered before-hand and tested for in the data analysis. These considerations along with exploratory data analysis techniques, define the scope of statistical analysis of case-control data.

6.3 CONCLUSION

It is obviously difficult to address all potential issues related to statistical analysis of data in case-control studies within the limits of a single chapter, but we believe that this chapter provides a solid initial step in planning and carrying out such analyses. We recommend the following further readings on this topic: Breslow and Day, 1980 for conceptually more in-depth discussion of analysis of case-control data (16), Hosmer and Lemeshow, 2000 for more applied topics (17), and Harrell, 2002 (18) for general issues related to statistical analysis of any data.

REFERENCES

1. Robins JM. Data, design, and background knowledge in etiologic inference. *Epidemiology*. 2001;11:313-320.
2. Diggle PJ, Liang K-Y, Zeger SL. *Analysis of Longitudinal Data*. New York: Oxford Science Publications; 1994.
3. Rubin DB. Inference and Missing Data. *Biometrika*. 1975;63(3):581-592.
4. Harrell FE. *Regression Modeling Strategies*, chapter 3, Missing data. pp. 41-52. New York: Springer-Verlag; 2002.
5. Hastie T, Tibshirani R. *Generalized Additive Models*. London: Chapman & Hall; 1990.
6. Weisskopf MG, O'Reilly E, Chen H, et al. Plasma urate and risk of Parkinson's disease. *Am J Epidemiol*. 2007;166 (5):561-567.
7. Becher H. General principles of data analysis: continuous covariables in epidemiologic studies, chapter II.2. In: Wolfgang Aherns, Iris Pigeot eds. *Handbook of Epidemiology*. Berlin: Springer, 2005:597-624.
8. Harrell FE. *Regression Modeling Strategies*, chapter 2, General Aspects of Fitting Regression Models. pp.16-26. New York: Springer-Verlag; 2002.
9. Rothman KJ, Greenland S. *Modern Epidemiology*, 2nd ed. Philadelphia: Lippincott-Raven; 1998.
10. Merchant AT, Pitiphat W. Directed acyclic graphs (DAGs): an aid to assess confounding in dental research. *Community Dent Oral Epidemiol*. 2002;30: 399-404.
11. Mantel N, Haenszel W. Statistical aspects of the analysis of data from retrospective studies of disease. *J Natl Cancer Inst*. 1959;22:719-748.

12. Hannibal CG, Rossing MA, Wicklund KG, Cushing-Haugen KL. Analgesic drug use and risk of epithelial ovarian cancer. *Am J Epidemiol*. 2008;167 (12): 1430-1437.

13. Moorman PG, Calingaert B, Palmieri RT, et al. Hormonal risk factors for ovarian cancer in premenopausal and postmenopausal women. *Am. J. Epidemiol*. 2008;167 (9):1059-1069.

14. McNemar Q. Note on the sampling error of the difference between correlated proportions or percentages. *Psychometrika*. 1947;12:153-157.

15. Hosmer DW, Lemeshow S. *Applied Logistic Regression*, 2nd ed, chapter 7: Logistic regression for matched case-control studies. New York: Wiley-Interscience; 2000: 223-259.

16. Breslow NE, Day NE. *Statistical Methods in Cancer Research, Volume I, The Analysis of Case-Control Studies*. Lyon: IARC Scientific Publications; 1980.

17. Hosmer DW, Lemeshow S. *Applied Logistic Regression*. New York: Wiley-Interscience; 2000.

18. Harrell FE. *Regression Modeling Strategies*. New York: Springer-Verlag; 2002.

7

APPLICATIONS: OUTBREAK INVESTIGATION

Haroutune K. Armenian

OUTLINE

This chapter aims to

1. describe the steps involved in a traditional outbreak investigation;
2. identify some of the problems with the traditional method of outbreak investigation;

3. highlight the advantages of the case-control method in outbreak investigation; and
4. provide guidelines for a case-control investigation of an outbreak.

7.1 OVERVIEW

7.1.1 *Definition*

An outbreak is a situation in the community where the observed occurrence of disease is in excess of normal expectancy.

Other terms used for outbreak include *epidemics* and *disease clusters*. According to this definition and in order to characterize an outbreak, we need to

1. *define* clearly the disease or outcome of interest;
2. *delimit the community* where the outbreak is occurring; and
3. *identify* what is the *"normal expectancy"* of the occurrence of the condition in the specified community.

A health center physician in Bahrain reported a case of relatively sudden enlargement of the breasts or gynecomastia in a 7-year-old prepubertal girl (1). Case finding from the same village revealed seven additional cases in children about the same age from the same village in a total of five households. The case-control investigation of this outbreak led to the potential source—the milk from a cow from the village that was receiving estrogen injections. In this particular situation, gynecomastia is very unusual as a condition in prepubertal children and our definition of the disease or the outcome is simple and is based on an anatomic feature. The community of interest is the village where these cases are occurring and can be very well delineated. One could assume, however, that the reference community in this particular situation could very well be the total population of Bahrain: with such a rare condition, we could consider it as an epidemic in the whole country.

Outbreaks may be identified in a number of ways, at all levels of the population, and the health-care system. The first reports of a possible outbreak could come from (1) individuals, bringing to the attention of the health department an unusual occurrence of three persons with diarrhea in their family following a common meal in a restaurant; (2) physicians, coming across an unexpected pattern of two cases of myalgia with eosinophilia in their practice; or, (3) epidemiologists, identifying an unexpected increase in the rates of influenza from routine surveillance reports.

Outbreaks are frequently at the center of public attention, which is why the epidemiologist's management of the situation is often closely scrutinized. Thus, early preparation for investigating outbreaks is critical.

Outbreaks result from a clustering of people with illness in time, place, and, on occasion, personal characteristics. Time-place clustering is not particular to outbreaks and may occur whenever confluence of cases occurs due to some common etiological characteristics or common exposure. What makes such clustering an outbreak, by definition, is that what is observed exceeds normal expectancy in a particular group. One of the functions of routine surveillance and monitoring of important health problems is early identification of such clustering of cases in the population. Current technology including Geographic Information Systems allows us to make such analyses of clustering a matter of routine and on an ongoing basis.

Our discussion on outbreaks in this chapter is not specific to infectious disease epidemics. The principles described here apply to all outcomes where an unusual cluster of cases may occur. We may have outbreaks or epidemics of suicide, toxic exposure, or as a result of disasters. The investigative methods of these latter situations will be similar to those we use for infectious disease outbreaks.

7.1.2 Circumstances Leading to an Outbreak

A number of circumstances may lead to an outbreak or epidemic. In most of these situations, an outbreak is the result of some ecologic imbalance between the host, the agent, and the environment. These circumstances include (2)

A change in the dosage or virulence of the agent that causes the disease. Influenza pandemics are typically caused by the introduction of a new strain of the virus in human populations. Similarly, over the past century the introduction of the El Tor strain of the cholera bacillus has been at the root of major epidemics of cholera that have spread globally from Asia to Africa and to South America.

The introduction of a new pathogen into the community. An example is the introduction of the HIV virus in the early 1980s that caused a wildfire of epidemics (3). Similarly, the introduction of measles and tuberculosis by colonists to indigenous populations has decimated these populations throughout the colonial periods.

The presence of a large number of people who are susceptible to the disease. Previous economic and political stressors created an environment in Armenia in the late 1980s where most people were susceptible to depression. Thus, a massive epidemic of depression and related psychopathologies followed the 1988 earthquake in northern Armenia. The development of modern irrigation canals in Egypt and other African countries has exposed new communities to Schistosomiasis, as previously these communities were spared exposure to the agent in the absence of a water distribution system for irrigation.

Host susceptibility and response. Effective therapeutic immunosuppression makes the host susceptible to the development of non-Hodgkins lymphomas, and a dramatic increase in these cancers has been observed in people undergoing such therapy for a variety of purposes.

New portals of entry for the agent. Epidemics of serum hepatitis were observed following the early introduction of blood transfusions.

The decision to investigate a reported outbreak is very much influenced by the resources available in the community, the severity of the outbreak in terms of numbers and nature of the condition (e.g., seriousness of morbidity, amount of disability it causes, and mortality), and the political and sociocultural expediencies.

7.1.3 *Features of an Outbreak Investigation*

Outbreak investigations have certain features that are uncommon in other epidemiologic studies or investigations:

1. In most of these outbreaks, we are dealing with an *urgent situation* where the epidemiologist cannot take an extended amount of time to plan the study, implement it, and develop a final report about it. Here, the epidemiologist needs to be well-trained professionally to plan the investigation—sometimes within hours—or use some standardized approaches that are preset for investigating such outbreaks.

2. In outbreaks, *decisions* will be made *at every step* of the investigation and sometimes on the basis of data that are not yet complete. The potential for making mistakes and for biases to mislead in such decisions can be very high.

3. The process of outbreak investigation may involve a number of *different approaches and designs* to explain the epidemic and to provide recommendations for intervention. To solve etiological relationships and understand methods of transmission, the epidemiologist may use a whole spectrum of investigative tools. These may include clinical examinations, environmental inspections, surveys of the cases and the population, special laboratory analyses, and nonconcurrent cohort studies, as well as case-control studies.

4. The process of such an investigation is very *dynamic* and we may need to introduce a great deal of flexibility in our search for

etiological factors. If necessary, the epidemiologist working on such an investigation will assess the situation continuously and redirect the investigation; this is often the case for an ongoing epidemic with changing trends.

5. The investigation is conducted with an objective of applying *prevention and control measures as soon as possible*. Thus, following initial data gathering, if we can identify some actions that will help control the outbreak, we may have to take these measures. There may be some simple interventions we can implement without having to wait until the whole investigative process is completed.

6. The outbreak investigation may have *multiple objectives*. We need to identify the *agent* causing the disease in affected individuals; we need to localize the *source* of the outbreak; and we need to determine the *mode of transmission* of the agent. Often we are aware of the agent that causes the disease through our clinical investigation and laboratory confirmation of the cases. We may know that we are dealing with cholera or a typhoid epidemic. The aim of the epidemiologist in such situations is to identify the source of the epidemic and its mode of transmission. A case-control approach is useful to tackle an investigation of an outbreak of unknown etiology as well as to elucidate the source and mechanism of transmission.

7. Although a small number of cases may limit the power of the test to find a causative factor, we may still embark on an investigation because of the *statutory authority* that requires that such an investigation be conducted. When numbers of cases are limited, alternative investigative procedures such as case investigations or case-series studies (Chapter 1) may be considered.

8. A number of other problems may mar the investigation of an outbreak, including the inability to conduct tests for laboratory investigation because of lack of either resources or *timely collection of specimens*.

There are a number of steps a well-trained and well-prepared epidemiologist needs to take to investigate any outbreak, including ensuring the availability of the necessary logistical support.

Prior to embarking on the detailed investigation, we need to confirm the existence of an epidemic. Preliminary reports of an outbreak or a cluster of cases may be misleading. We need first to validate the diagnosis or clinical presentation of the reported cases and then to assess whether the observation of this cluster is unusual with regard to time, place, and persons. These initial cases may undergo preliminary interviews to identify some common characteristics. This step may help to identify the population base from which these cases came and to develop some preliminary hypotheses about the potential etiologies or common sources of exposure.

Our investigation will be incomplete if we do not make an intensive effort at finding additional cases based on a preliminary case definition. Thus, a defined population at risk is critical at this step. All potential sources of case identification need to be surveyed to detect cases not previously reported.

A distribution of cases by *time* can provide information on the nature of the outbreak—whether we are dealing with a protracted outbreak or common source outbreaks. Case clustering by *geography* will allow us to further explore the importance of geographic characteristics in this outbreak. Based on such an initial review of descriptive epidemiological data, one may develop hypotheses that can be pursued in an analytic study. Deciding the next step of the investigation is based on our ability to define as well as enumerate the base population where the outbreak started. Outbreaks that occur in a well-defined group, such as a cohort, should be investigated and analyzed using the traditional retrospective cohort approach where we compare individuals exposed to the suspected agent and persons who are not. An outbreak that is diffuse, and where it is not possible to enumerate the base cohort or exposed population, is a candidate for a case-control investigation.

7.2 TRADITIONAL COHORT-BASED INVESTIGATION

7.2.1 Overview

The traditional outbreak investigation is based on a method of comparison of the incidence-attack rate of the disease in persons exposed to the suspected agent (or agents) to the incidence-attack rate of the disease in persons not exposed to the suspected agent. Thus, the factor for which the difference in incidence between exposed and nonexposed is maximized is judged as the cause of the outbreak.

As judgment in such a traditional analysis is based on our ability to calculate incidence rates, we need to be able to count a denominator for the exposed group and a denominator for the nonexposed group. This is an important conceptual and operational shortcoming of the traditional approach of outbreak investigation. When the cohort or base population is easy to identify and enumerate, such as a church group charity luncheon or an outbreak on a cruise ship, this traditional approach is preferred.

Between November 10 and 13, 1990, 42 people attended a cake decorating conference in Michigan. On November 12th, 25 cases of diarrheal illness in the conference participants were reported to the local health department. Questionnaires were distributed to all conference attendees on the same day requesting information about symptoms, time of onset, food items consumed for the three preceding days, and illness in the family. A case of illness was defined as a conference attendee with acute diarrhea, stomach cramps, and nausea or unusual flatulence. A total of 32 attendees met the case definition. Two food items served at lunch on the second day of the conference were associated with an increased risk of illness: minestrone soup (relative risk 4.92, 95% CI 1.23–infinity) and fettuccini Alfredo (relative risk 3.26, 95% CI 0.59–17.94). Eleven stool specimens obtained from twelve ill persons had greater than 10^5 Clostridium perfringens spores per gram of feces (4).

7.2.2 Model

The model of a traditional outbreak investigation has been structured in the first half of the 20th century and Wade Hampton Frost, the first professor of epidemiology in the United States, was one of the first to introduce it to the classroom. The steps in the investigation of such an outbreak involve

1. problem definition. Is there an epidemic?
2. orientation of the epidemic as to time, place, and persons. Study time of onset and epidemic curve, review the geographic distribution of the cases (spot maps), and identify common personal characteristics of the cases. At this stage one may attempt to calculate attack rates by various characteristics if crude denominators are available.
3. Formulation of a hypothesis (es) based on a review of the data as per above.
4. Testing the hypothesis. The investigator is asked to identify further cases of the epidemic at this stage, and do laboratory tests on the etiology and the particular sero-epidemiological characteristics of the agent. At this stage, and if it was possible to identify the baseline population where the exposure(s) occurred, it is recommended to conduct an attack-rate based analysis of the data.
5. Make the inferences about the epidemic and the appropriate recommendations in a report.

7.3 INDICATIONS FOR USING THE CASE-CONTROL APPROACH IN OUTBREAK INVESTIGATION

As stated earlier the major indication for using the case-control method in outbreaks is the difficulty of enumerating a base population or a cohort with a countable denominator for the exposed and unexposed groups. Some more specific indications for the use of the case-control method in outbreak investigation include (5)

Subgroup analysis. There may be situations where the enumeration of the full cohort is possible but due to a limitation of resources one may decide to consider a case-control *analysis in a subgroup* of the cohort. An example of such a situation—the 2004 Zambia cholera epidemic investigation—is presented in the next section.

Exploratory analysis. In a major epidemic with large numbers of cases, it may be best to do a quick case-control analysis with an initial group of cases and healthy controls to orient the full investigation of the large cohort. Such an analysis of cases and controls is primarily *exploratory* for potential factors that may be involved in this epidemic.

Impossibility of enumeration of base population. Where an enumeration of the base population or the cohort is not possible, the analytic options may be limited to the case-control method.

Test of specific hypothesis in a subgroup. In a number of outbreak investigations, one may decide to focus on a *specific hypothesis* that can be *tested in a subgroup.* If, for example, in the broader study it is identified that exposure to a widely used product is the risk factor for the disease, then in a further analysis, one may choose to answer the question of why the vast majority of people using the product do not develop the disease. A case-control analysis where both the cases and controls are users of the product may lead to the answer of the more specific question of method of transmission of agent in this population.

7.4 EXAMPLES OF OUTBREAKS USING THE CASE-CONTROL METHOD

In a study of the use of the case-control method for outbreak investigation, Fonseca and Armenian (6) observed the paucity of published case-control investigations of outbreaks prior to the 1970s. Currently a vast majority of outbreaks are investigated using the case-control method, and below is a sample of some of these investigations of outbreaks, along with a discussion of some of their problems.

7.4.1 Legionnaire's Disease

One of the earliest case-control investigations of an outbreak was the major epidemic of Legionnaire's disease in 1976 in Philadelphia (7). This was a new infectious disease of unknown etiology that was expressed in an explosive outbreak of pneumonia with 28 fatal cases out of 182 initially reported cases. Because the common thread of most of these cases was their presence at the 1976 American Legion Convention in Philadelphia, the unknown disease was named Legionnaire's Disease. A case was defined as a patient with fever, radiologic evidence of pneumonia, and presence at the convention site. A number of unexplained cases of pneumonia occurring simultaneously in Philadelphia with no contact with the convention were termed Bond Street pneumonia, after the address where the convention was held. Eight different surveys were conducted to investigate this epidemic, including two case-control "surveys."

Through these surveys the investigators were able to calculate various attack rates of the disease in the different subcategories of hotel personnel and the participants of the convention with the highest attack rates occurring among the convention participants. Using a crude case-control analysis the investigators developed a high index of suspicion for the use of the water fountains at the hotel where the convention was held; the new agent for the disease was later identified from the water tanks. Of the 69 cases studied in one of the case-control studies, 65% drank water from the hotel system, while only 48% of 976 well delegates drank such water (OR = 2.0, 95% CI 1.2–3.4).

A number of problems are evident in the two case-control studies of this investigation, including inappropriate design and analytic techniques.

7.4.2 Toxic-Shock Syndrome

Sudden onset of disease with high fever, headache, sore throat, diarrhea, renal failure, and sudden onset refractory hypotension characterized this toxic-shock syndrome epidemic (8). To identify cases, 3,500 practitioners in Wisconsin were mailed questionnaires. The practitioners reporting a case of the disease were then asked to select from the same practice three controls without the disease matched to the cases for menstruation status and for age within two years. Cases were interviewed by one of the authors, although the authors do not specify the person(s) interviewing the controls. Some of the problems with this investigation include control selection, interviewing, and analysis.

7.4.3 Asthma Deaths in New Zealand

Epidemics of asthma deaths have been reported from a number of countries since the 1970s. Rea and colleagues wanted to elucidate the etiology of such an outbreak in New Zealand (9). This was a population-based case-control study with two control groups. All deaths in people less than 60 years in the Auckland population, possibly due to asthma, over a two-year period were investigated as cases. Over the study period, the authors identified 44 deaths in Auckland with reversible airway obstruction. Two controls were selected per case, a hospital control and a community-based control. A different interviewer interviewed the community controls. Problems with this study included recall bias (dead cases), as well as different interviewers for the two control groups.

7.4.4 School Outbreak of a Psychogenic Illness

A total of 65 students and one teacher reported symptoms of dizziness, chills, nausea, headache, difficulty in breathing, and fainting over a 24-hour period in a school in Singapore caused by an "alleged exposure" to a gas in the school. Extensive environmental investigations did not reveal any such sources of gas exposure. Goh and colleagues conducted a case-control study comparing all the affected students to an equal number of unaffected student controls from the same classrooms, and from the same ethnicity and gender as the cases (10). Detailed and systematic interviewing of the cases and controls did not reveal any differences as to suspected exposures between the two groups.

7.4.5 Reye Syndrome

Reye Syndrome (RS) is a neurological condition with encephalopathy for a majority of the cases. It was first reported in 1963 in Australia and the United States. A number of outbreaks of RS were described in the United States associated with outbreaks of influenza and other viral infections, and case fatality rates of up to 40% were reported initially. The possibility of an association between RS and aspirin was suggested but was not readily accepted because aspirin was such a commonly used medication in all such viral infections. Three case-control studies were conducted in Arizona, Ohio, and Michigan to test this hypothesis (11).

Between December 1978 and March 1980, the Ohio State Department of Health prospectively identified 159 cases of RS from 6 pediatrics centers in the state. Most of these cases were identified during epidemics of influenza or had antecedent varicella during that period. Controls were selected from the same classrooms or neighborhoods as the cases and were matched to the cases for age, gender, race, and the occurrence of a similar antecedent illness within one week of that which occurred in the case. Cases and controls were interviewed about the use of medications following the viral infection but prior to the onset of the RS. A multiple logistic regression analysis with fever, headache, aspirin intake, and sore throat in the model, estimated the relative risk of taking aspirin for RS at 11.3 (95% CI 2.7–47.5). Other medications like acetaminophen did not show such case-control differences.

A number of potential problems were highlighted when these case-control studies were conducted, including (1) differential recall of medication intake between cases and controls when cases suffered a more severe condition; and (2) the potential that cases had a more severe form of the original viral disease that resulted in their taking more medications. Both initial and subsequent analyses addressed these potential issues. The fact that there was no association with acetaminophen—an analgesic-antipyretic very frequently used for these viral infections—speaks against recall bias, and adjustments for disease severity in the various models did not alter the direction or the size of the association with aspirin.

Following a number of reviews and audits of the data from these case-control studies, the CDC and the FDA issued warnings and recommendations about the use of aspirin in children with influenza and other viral infections such as chickenpox. A Public Health Task Force designed a new nationwide case-control study with a pilot study that confirmed an odds ratio of 16.1 for the association with aspirin. The larger study could not be completed because of the lack of cases of RS in subsequent years in the 33 pediatric tertiary care centers that were involved in this study. This probably reflected the declining incidence of RS following the application of the recommendations by the CDC and the FDA regarding aspirin use in children for influenza and chickenpox (11).

7.4.6 Cholera Epidemic in Lusaka, Zambia

Zambia has had major epidemics of El Tor cholera between 1991 and 2004, with the earlier epidemics affecting over 10,000 persons. Between November 2003 and January 2004, an estimated 2,500 cholera cases and 128 deaths from cholera were reported in Lusaka, the capital city. A case-control study was initiated to identify the source of the cholera and its method of transmission. A total of 71 case-control pairs were enrolled in the study, and consumption of raw vegetables was associated with cholera (matched odds ratio = 3.9; 95% CI = 1.7–9.6) (12). Presence of hand soap at home was considered a proxy for hand washing and was protective from cholera (OR = 0.14, 95% CI 0.05–0.40). Water treatment and chlorination at home was used to the same extent for cases and controls. The investigators highlighted that the primary mode of transmission in this epidemic was food borne, and recommendations focused primarily on this finding.

7.5 ADVANTAGES OF THE CASE-CONTROL METHOD IN OUTBREAK INVESTIGATION

Based on the above examples of outbreaks investigated using the case-control method, the advantages of the case-control method compared to the traditional approaches can be listed as follows:

1. In an outbreak we must identify an etiology or its mode of transmission from a number of possibilities. The case-control method is well suited to *study multiple etiologic hypotheses* and their interactions.
2. In a case-control investigation of an outbreak, it is not necessary to identify a population base to study exposure–outcome relationships. A case-control investigation of an outbreak can be set up even *when our base population cannot be completely enumerated* or defined.
3. The case-control method *does not have to exclude any cases* of the disease because of a preliminary incomplete definition of the epidemic's location.
4. The case-control method allows us to conduct an *analysis of interactions* between suspected etiologic factors and it can control all forms of confounding effectively in a multivariate analysis.
5. Within hours of the reporting of the outbreak one may be able to design and implement a case-control investigation and provide the results of the analysis within a few days, which denotes *efficiency*.

7.6 GUIDELINES FOR USING THE CASE-CONTROL METHOD FOR OUTBREAK INVESTIGATION

7.6.1 *Case Definition and Selection*

As stated earlier (Chapter 2), case definition is very much dependent on a clear delineation of the problem or the epidemic. The epidemic needs to be delineated along the three parameters of time, place, and persons, and it is also essential that we have a clear clinical characterization of the cases. To develop such a case definition, we may review the original cases (case-series) reported for investigation and devise a preliminary case definition based on the common characteristics of these initial cases. Thus, for example, these common characteristics may be that all reported cases are members of a club or are employed by the same company. As a result, we may decide to include membership in the club or employment with the company as part of our preliminary case definition. However, if we are not certain that our outbreak is limited to this subgroup, we may decide to keep a broad case definition without incorporating any common epidemiological parameters. In the latter situation, and as our investigation progresses, we may decide to revisit our case definition and make it more specific as we observe common characteristics.

Following our initial review of the cases, and having a reasonable definition, we need to move next to identifying as many of the cases from the epidemic as possible. The search for additional cases may involve a number of sources including various health-care delivery facilities, diagnostic laboratories, and passive surveillance systems, as well as conducting active surveillance. If our definition is too specific, then we may decide to use two or more categories of cases. Persons fulfilling all the criteria for case definition may be classified as *definite*, while those having missing data on certain elements of our case definition may be classified as *probable*.

7.6.2 Control Definition and Selection

As in other case-control studies, controls in outbreak investigations need to come from the same base population as the cases: the controls need to come from people without the disease, selected from the cohort or group where the outbreak is being studied or where it is circumscribed.

Identifying the base population or the cohort where the outbreak has occurred may be critical to the selection of the number of controls and process of identifying them. At times over half of the group at risk of exposure may develop the disease and we may end up with very few eligible controls. When we are not able to enumerate a base cohort for the outbreak, we may try to select controls from the same sources where the cases are identified. Thus, if cases were identified through laboratory reports, then our controls may be identified from the same laboratory records from persons who do not have the disease under investigation.

During our investigation of an outbreak, as our hypothesis becomes better defined and focused, we need to revisit the appropriateness of our control group. As our understanding of etiology evolves from a broader association to a search for more specific mechanisms, we may use controls that are exposed to the general factor. Thus, in an investigation of the eosinophilia-myalgia syndrome (13), the authors used three different levels of case-control analysis: first they identified that patients taking L-tryptophan (L-T) were at risk of developing the disease. At a second level, they asked why the vast majority of L-T users did not develop the disease: this query led to a case-control analysis where both the cases and controls were L-T users. This second level of analysis identified one brand of L-T as the culprit. As this brand of L-T had been in use for many years causing no such illness, the investigators pushed their analysis further, comparing cases and controls who were users of this same brand of L-T. As a result they were able to identify a particular batch of L-T whereby the manufacturing process had been altered.

7.6.3 Measurement of Exposure

Information about exposure in an outbreak can be collected from a variety of sources. The most common approach is usually through interviewing cases and controls or a sample of the population at risk as to the use or ingestion of various suspected factors that may cause the disease. It is also important for most investigations to test samples of food and other material for the suspected agent. Thus, evidence is gathered at multiple levels to confirm or disprove our hypothesized etiology (ies). As in other questionnaire-based investigations, recall may be a major problem. In a simulated outbreak, where a potluck lunch was videotaped, the investigators collected exposure information 50 to 69 hours after the lunch, with misclassification of exposure occurring in both directions. Among participants 32 failed to report 58 items that they actually consumed and reported consuming 24 items that they had not. Only 12.5% of the participants made no errors in reporting what they had consumed

Often there may be more intensive efforts at generating exposure information in cases than in controls. The cases may have been interviewed by their physicians and the field epidemiologists prior to being formally interviewed by the staff. Thus, differential recall between cases and controls is sometimes a real possibility. The interviewers may be fully aware of the case-control status, which may also potentially bias the results.

7.6.4 Biases

As stated previously, the lack of independence of the two processes of identifying and selecting cases and controls and of gathering information about exposure will lead to biases. Misclassification can result at the level of case-control selection when some of the controls are subclinical cases.

7.6.5 Serial Case-Control Studies

Sometimes it may not be possible to identify the exact mechanisms of transmission and source of the exposure within one case-control study. As in the investigation of the eosinophilia-myalgia syndrome described above three levels of case-control analyses were conducted to identify the specific source and mode of transmission of the exposure.

Similarly, Llewellyn et al. used two sequential case-control studies to investigate an outbreak of salmonellosis in Wales (14). The first level of the case-control study identified an association between the illness and eating ham (OR 4.50, 95% CI 1.10–21.8). Cases were persons with the illness and controls were selected from the same general practice without the illness. A second case-control analysis was conducted whereby both cases and controls had consumed ham to obtain detailed information about the sources of the ham and its preparation and storage. This second case-control study identified a single common ham producer as the source the outbreak (OR 25.0, 95% CI 2.33–1, 155).

7.7 CASE-CONTROL INVESTIGATION AS PART OF AN ONGOING SURVEILLANCE SYSTEM AND OTHER NOTES

It is possible to develop an ongoing case-control analysis as part of an ongoing disease surveillance system. Most disease surveillance systems collect data on the occurrence of the reportable conditions and analyze them on a periodic basis for trends and case characteristics. If we develop a system whereby as the cases are reported and investigated, similar data are collected from a nondiseased control on a regular basis, the series of cases of reported disease could be compared to the series of nondiseased controls and potential sources of ongoing exposure identified. Such a system would allow taking preventive action prior to the occurrence of a major epidemic.

In an outbreak, we are pressed for time, and a rapid end to the investigation may be critical to preventing new cases. Thus, a sequential approach to sampling cases and controls and analyzing data on a periodic basis will allow us to identify etiologic relationships as early as possible and to intervene on a timely basis. A sequential approach to data analysis will also help us to assess false leads to etiology and modify our data collection instruments accordingly. This approach assumes that we have no significant variation across time of the characteristics of the cases and controls, as well as the exposure patterns. A simple test of constancy of these characteristics can be conducted by comparing cases and controls at various time periods.

In any outbreak, it is important to conduct a separate in-depth case investigation of any *unusual cases* that do not fit the general pattern. The information yield of such unusual cases may be very high compared to the other cases. For example, in trying to determine why one female case occurs in an epidemic of otherwise all male cases may allow us to identify the fact that this only female case was the wife of one of the cases and she shared one particular type of food that the husband brought home following dinner at an all-male club.

A frequent mistake in many outbreak investigations is obtaining specimens for laboratory examination and testing too late; this could include, for example, that the suspected foods have been thrown away or the effects of the disease have waned. Thus, prior to conducting your case-control or other type of investigation, plan for the entire range of specimens that you need to gather and obtain them from the subjects or the sources of suspected exposure. In the previously cited outbreak of gynecomastia in prepubertal children in Bahrain, the investigators were late by two weeks to collect specimen from the children and the cow to conduct estrogen measurements. By the time such specimen were collected the clinical picture in the children had returned to normal and the cow had disappeared.

Finally, an investigator needs to be concerned about latency. Once the disease is identified, it is possible to get a clear idea about its incubation period. Thus, your case-control investigation of exposures can focus on the period of time that is located appropriately within the period of latency of that disease.

REFERENCES

1. Kimball AM, Hamadeh R, Mahmood RA, et al. Gynaecomastia among children in Bahrain. *Lancet*. 1981;21;1(8221):671-672.
2. Kelsey JL, Whittemore AS, Evans AS, Thompson WD. *Methods in Observational Epidemiology*. 2nd ed. New York: Oxford University Press; 1996: 270-272.
3. Jaffe HW, Choi K, Thomas PA, et al. National case-control study of Kaposi's sarcoma and *Pneumocystis carinii*. Pneumonia in homosexual men: Part 1, epidemiologic results. *Ann Intern Med*. 1983;99:145-151.
4. Roach RL, Sienko DG. Clostridium perfringens outbreak associated with minestrone soup. *Am J Epidemiol*. 1992;136:1288-1291.
5. Dwyer DM, Strickler H, Goodman RA, Armenian HK. Use of the case-control studies in outbreak investigations. *Epidemiol Rev*. 1994;16:109-123.
6. Fonseca MG, Armenian HK. Use of the case-control method in outbreak investigations. *Am J Epidemiol*. 1991 Apr 1;133(7):748-752.
7. Fraser DW, Tsai TR, Orenstein W, et al. Legionnaires' disease. Description of an epidemic of pneumonia. *N Engl J Med*. 1977;297:1189-1197.
8. Davis JP, Chesney PJ, Wand PJ, LaVenture M. Toxic-shock syndrome. *N Engl J Med*. 1980;303:1429-1435.
9. Rea HH, Scragg R, Jackson R, Beaglehole R, Fenwick J, Sutherland DC. A case-control study of deaths from asthma. *Thorax*. 1986;41:833-839.

10. Goh KT. Epidemiological enquiries into a school outbreak of an unusual illness. *Int J Epidemiol*. 1987;16:265-270.
11. CDC. Reye syndrome. *MMWR*. 1997;46:750-755.
12. CDC. Cholera epidemic associated with raw vegetables – Lusaka, Zambia, 2003–2004. *MMWR*. 2004;53:783-786.
13. Belongia EA, Hedberg CW, Gleich GJ, et al. An investigation of the cause of the eosinophilia-myalgia syndrome associated with tryptophan use.*N Engl J Med*. 1990 Aug 9;323(6):357-365.
14. Llewellyn LJ, Evans MR, Palmer SR. Use of sequential case-control studies to investigate a community salmonella outbreak in Wales. *J Epidemiol Community Health*. 1998;52:272-276.

8

GENETIC EPIDEMIOLOGY FOR CASE-BASED DESIGNS

M. Daniele Fallin and W.H. Linda Kao

OUTLINE

8.1 INTRODUCTION

Genetic epidemiology is one of the most rapidly growing fields of epidemiologic research. Almost every human disease has some genetic component, from disorders such as cystic fibrosis which are caused by specific genetic mutations, to complex diseases such as type 2 diabetes, which result from combinations of genes and/or exposures and lifestyles, to infectious diseases such as AIDS, which require an infectious agent, but where host immune-response is influenced by genes. For these reasons, almost all aspects of epidemiology require some knowledge of the use of genes as exposure variables in study design and analysis. This chapter will introduce the field of genetic epidemiology in general, then describe the unique aspects of considering genes as risk factors in an epidemiological study, and finally focus on designs and analysis strategies that use case sampling approaches to evaluate the influence of genes on disease risk. Two main designs will be highlighted: (1) the case-control design in which unrelated controls are sampled for comparison, and (2) the case-parent trio design in which parental genotypes are used as matched genetic controls. Design considerations and analytic methods are described for each. Options for evaluating gene–environment interactions are given within each design, and the particular utility of the case-only design for this purpose is discussed as well.

The main purpose of genetic epidemiology is to identify genes that cause, or contribute to risk for, human disease. The central paradigm for the identification of genes that contribute to disease risk involves a set of questions and design/analytic strategies to answer those questions (see Figure 8.1). First, there must be evidence that some proportion of disease variation or risk is due to genes. This can be addressed through migration, familial aggregation, adoption and twin studies, which aim to assess the heritability (the proportion of the phenotypic variation that is due to additive genetic effect) of the disease. One may also want to assess whether a particular risk model fits the disease patterns well. Such studies are usually based on disease patterns among families, using a methodology called segregation analysis.

Once a genetic component to disease has been established, the challenge becomes the identification of particular genes and gene variations that cause or increase risk for the disease. These studies are usually dichotomized, according to the design and type of genetic properties exploited by that design, into studies for genetic linkage analyses and studies for genetic association analyses. Both of these employ marker-based approaches (referred to as indirect genetic analyses), while genetic association studies also encompass the study of candidate variants with

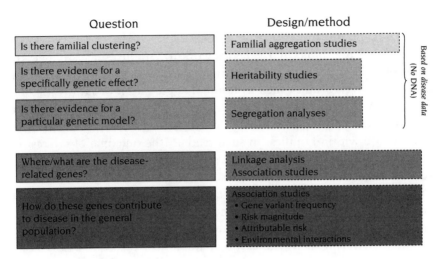

Figure 8.1. Central Paradigm for Genetic Epidemiology Research

previously known or hypothesized function, referred to as direct genetic analyses. Each of these questions and design options are important aspects of genetic epidemiology, but the focus of this chapter will be restricted to applications when sampling on case status, which include familial aggregation studies (no DNA required) and genetic association studies (direct or indirect genetic analyses).

The three most common designs using case-based sampling in genetic epidemiology are (1) the case-control design, where cases and representative controls from the same source sampling frame are included, (2) the case-parent trio design, where cases and their parents are sampled, and (3) case-only designs for questions regarding gene–environment or gene–gene interactions or for questions regarding response to treatment or interventions and genetic influences on prognosis, or natural history of disease. This chapter focuses on each of these three designs in turn, offering a paradigm for constructing the question, assessing the case characteristics, choosing an appropriate design, choosing appropriate exposures to measure, and analyzing the data collected. For each design, the outcome and genetic exposure variables will be defined, then the analytic methods for that design will be presented with examples, and finally, particular issues relevant to each design will be discussed.

8.2 TYPES OF GENETIC "EXPOSURE" VARIABLES

It is important to understand that different types of genetic information can be used in genetic epidemiology studies. In general, this information can be dichotomized into unmeasured versus measured genotypes. Before embarking on a genetics study that requires collection of DNA and molecular genetics work to establish measured genotypes of individuals, one should be convinced that genes play a role in disease etiology. Studies such as familial aggregation or family history studies, do not directly measure genotypes, but rather aim to establish evidence of a genetic component to etiology by assessing the clustering of a disease within families. In such studies, the outcome of interest is whether a person is affected with a particular disease, while the exposure of interest is whether the person had a family member with the same disease. This type of genetic "exposure" definition is discussed in Section 8.2.1 below. The bulk of genetic epidemiology studies, however, are concerned with relating measured genotypes of individuals to risk for disease. What exactly is measured, and how it is used to assess association, is an important decision point for design, and requires a basic understanding of the terminology and motivation for different types of genetic studies. Section 8.2.2 will describe different types of genetic polymorphisms, how they are measured, and how these measurements define exposure for the three study designs described in this chapter.

8.2.1 *Family History*

One of the main hypotheses in genetic epidemiology is whether the disease clusters in families. This is necessary, but insufficient, to infer genetic etiology of disease. One way to address this hypothesis is to employ the classic case-control design where cases and controls are compared with respect to disease status of their relatives. In this setting, the exposure is family history of disease, which may simply be a dichotomized variable indicating presence or absence of other family members with disease, or may be extended to specify different levels of family history, according to degree of relationship between the participant and the affected family member, or may be summarized as a family history score, which calculates the excess risk of disease among all family members given their expected disease risk. This approach has the advantage of characterizing the overall burden of disease in the family and has been used previously to determine whether family history of coronary heart disease is associated with plasma levels of hemostatic factors (1).

However, most studies may not have collected complete disease information in all 1st- or 2nd-degree relatives. More often, information on parental history of disease is available, which may simply be characterized as a dichotomized variable. Using the dichotomized family history variable, familial aggregation is supported if the odds of cases

Table 8.1. Exposure Defined by Family History

Retrospective			
Exposure	*Outcome*		
Family History	Cases	Controls	*Odds Ratio*
Present	*a*	*b*	*(a/c)/(b/d) = ad/bc*
Absent	*c*	*d*	*1*
Prospective			
Exposure	*Outcome*		
Relative of a:	Affected	Not affected	*Relative's Relative Risk*
Case	*a*	*b*	*a/(a + b)/*
			c/(c + d)
Control	*c*	*d*	*1*

having at least one affected relative is greater than the odds of controls having affected relatives (see Table 8.1, top panel).

Two potential drawbacks of comparing cases and controls with respect to the dichotomized family history of disease are that family history is a function of both risk and family size and risk factors of the relatives are not accounted for in this type of analysis. Therefore, an alternative way to approach familial aggregation is to consider family members of cases and controls as the exposed and unexposed individuals, respectively, and assess their disease occurrence prospectively (see Table 8.1, bottom panel). This can provide an estimate of the risk to relatives of cases (exposed group) versus risk to relatives of controls (unexposed). The risk to relatives of cases is sometimes called a "recurrence risk," and can be specific to a particular type of relationship. For example, if siblings of cases were considered as the exposed group, the incidence of disease among these siblings could be used to establish the "sibling recurrence risk." The ratio of this sibling recurrence risk to the risk of disease in the general population is the "sibling relative risk," often denoted λs in genetics literature.

Although this is a useful assessment of the potential genetic component of disease risk, there are several caveats to interpretation. One main consideration is the multiple methods to assess family history of disease, which can lead to large differences in how this "exposure" variable is measured across studies, and how an association should be interpreted. While the most basic family history information characterizes disease status of parents, of siblings, or of any 1st-degree relative, more detailed family history may be extended to include multiple relatives of different types, and multiple criterion for considering a relative "affected." The most important caveat for interpreting a relationship between disease risk and family history as an "exposure" is the fact that familial clustering of disease can be due also to shared family environmental risk factors. Further studies that can specifically estimate heritability by parsing environmental and genetic contributions to the similarity between family members, such as twin studies, are necessary to confirm a genetic component to disease risk (2). In summary, case-control studies are often already designed to address nongenetic risk factors, and the addition of a well-designed family history exposure variable can be very useful in addressing the potential genetic component to etiology before undertaking a measured genotype study.

8.2.2 Measured Genotypes

The bulk of genetic studies in epidemiology rely on measured genotypes as exposures of interest. These require collection of DNA samples and molecular genetic analysis of particular genetic patterns in each participant. Before discussing the details of study designs that employ measured genotypes as exposures, it is important to define some basic terms of molecular genetics, and some common types of genotype measurements in epidemiology.

8.2.2.1 *Definition of terms.* The basic structural concepts in genetics are depicted in Figure 8.2. A gene is the physical entity transmitted from parent to offspring in reproduction that influences hereditary traits. Each gene contains a sequence of nucleotides (A,C,T or G for adenine, cytosine, thymine, and guanine, respectively) that encode the directions to create a particular protein product that has a function in the body. A chromosome is an arrangement of genes in linear order along microscopic threadlike bodies and may contain several thousand genes. The human genome has 22 unique chromosomes, in addition to the two sex chromosomes, X or Y. However, diploid organisms, such as humans, contain two copies of each type of chromosome, one inherited from the mother and the other from the father, resulting in 46 total chromosomes that make up the entire genome of an individual—44 autosomes, and two sex chromosomes. A locus corresponds to a location along a molecule of DNA. While every human being carries almost entirely identical sequences along the entire human genome, there are some areas where the genetic sequence is considered polymorphic, because more than one form, or sequence, can occur at the same locus across individuals. This locus is often termed a polymorphism, and there are several types of polymorphisms, as described in the next section. The particular sequence that defines different forms is often termed an allele, and any human carries two alleles at any locus (one from the father and one from the mother). In Figure 8.2, there are two types of alleles at

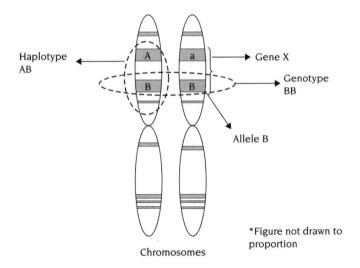

Figure 8.2. Relatioship between Genes, Alleles, Genotypes, and Diplotypes

locus A (allele "A" and allele "a") but only one type of allele at *locus B* (allele "B"). An individual's genotype is the combination of two alleles at any locus in the chromosome. If an individual's genotype contains two identical alleles, then that person is homozygous at that locus (e.g., Figure 8.2 shows a homozygous genotype at locus B). If an individual's two alleles are different, then that person is heterozygous at that locus (e.g., locus A in Figure 8.2).

8.2.2.2 *Genetic polymorphisms.* There are three common classes of genetic polymorphisms in the human genome: single nucleotide polymorphisms (SNPs), insertion/deletions, and duplications (see Figure 8.3). SNPs are common, but minute, alterations of a single nucleotide that occur in human DNA at a frequency of about one every 1,000 bases. Although many SNPs have no effect on cellular function, others may directly predispose people to disease or influence their response to a drug. SNPs are abundant, stable, widely distributed across the genome, and lend themselves to automated analysis on a very large scale. Finally, most SNPs are biallelic, that is, the polymorphism is one of two nucleotides. Insertion/deletions are a type of chromosomal abnormality in which a DNA sequence, either one or multiple nucleotides, is either inserted into, or deleted from, a genetic sequence, which can disrupt the normal structure and function of a gene. Duplications, often called microsatellites, are short sequences of DNA (usually one to 1,000 nucleotides) that are repeated multiple times. Microsatellites are widely distributed across the genome and are highly polymorphic, such that many different repeated

> **Single nucleotide polymorphism**
>   ❖ One nucleotide is replaced with
>   another.
>   ❖ Types of markers for studies:
>   SNPs, RFLP

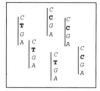

> **Deletion/Insertion**
>   ❖ Some chromosomes have a section
>   of sequence missing or inserted
>   ❖ Can be any size
>   ❖ Types of markers for studies:
>   *Insertion/deletion*

> **Duplication**
>   ❖ Like an insertion, usually tandem
>   repeats
>   ❖ Can be any size
>   ❖ Types of markers for studies:
>   STRs, *microsatellites*, VNTR

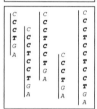

Figure 8.3. Common Types of Polymorphism in the Human Genome

lengths exist at the same location from person to person. Although they are another important and commonly studied class of genetic markers, this chapter will focus on SNPs to illustrate measured genotypes as the exposure of interest.

8.2.2.3 Relationship of alleles to genotypes (Hardy–Weinberg Principle). Alleles define the particular type, or category, of a polymorphic locus. As mentioned earlier, each human has two alleles, one per chromosome inherited from each parent. Thus, in a sample of $N = 100$ people, for any given locus there are 200 (2N) alleles. Genotypes, in contrast, are defined as the particular pairing of alleles at any locus carried by an individual. Therefore, in a sample of $N = 100$ people, there are 100 genotypes. Traditionally, human geneticists have characterized populations by allele frequencies, dividing the number of copies of a particular allele over the total number of chromosomes in the population (i.e., 2N chromosomes). Genotypes (allele pairs) are the observed genetic measure in most studies, and genotype frequencies can be estimated for any population by dividing the number of people with a particular genotype in a sample over the total number of people in the sample. Genotype and allele frequencies are closely related concepts, and under the assumption of a randomly mating population, they can be related to each other mathematically by assuming that homozygote genotype frequencies are equal to the square of the underlying allele frequency, and that heterozygote genotype frequencies are equal to twice the product of the underlying allele frequencies: $p(AA) = p^2$; $p(Aa) = 2pq$; $P(aa) = q^2$, where p is the frequency of allele A, q is the frequency of allele a, $P(AA)$ is the frequency of genotype AA, $P(Aa)$ is the frequency of genotype Aa, and $P(aa)$ is the frequency of genotype aa. This is the Hardy–Weinberg principle (HWP; also known as Hardy–Weinberg equilibrium (HWE), or Hardy–Weinberg law).

8.2.2.4 Relationship between alleles at separate loci (linkage equilibrium). In contrast to an allele, a haplotype defines the set of alleles on a chromosome that are in such close proximity that they are usually inherited as a unit. In Figure 8.2, alleles A and B define the haplotype AB on the left chromosome, while alleles a and B define haplotype aB on the other chromosome. The pair of haplotypes carried by one individual is considered a diplotype. Therefore, an allele at one locus is analogous to a haplotype across several loci, while a genotype at one locus is analogous to a diplotype across several loci. Just like the relationship between alleles and genotypes, the relationship between haplotypes and diplotypes at the population level can be defined mathematically, assuming HWP, such that a homozygote diplotype frequency should equal the square of the underlying haplotype's frequency, and a heterozygotes diplotype frequency should equal twice the product of the two underlying haplotype frequencies.

The concept of a haplotype has become an important unit for defining exposure in genetic epidemiology because it contains more information than an allele of a single locus. This is related to how haplotypes are distributed in a population. Under the Mendelian law of independent assortment, alleles at separate loci should be transmitted to a gamete independently. Therefore, there should be no relationship between the allelic status of a chromosome at locus A versus locus B. If this is true, then the frequency of any haplotype (for example AB, Ab, aB, or ab) should be predicted solely by the allele frequencies of those loci: $P(AB) = p_A p_B$; $P(Ab) = p_A q_B$; $P(aB) = q_A p_B$; $P(ab) = q_A q_B$, where p_A and q_A are frequencies of allele A and allele a, respectively, at locus A, and p_B and q_B are frequencies of allele B and allele b, respectively, at locus B. This situation is termed linkage equilibrium, because under equilibrium, alleles at separate loci assort together at random on a chromosome. However, for alleles located very close together on the same chromosome, this property does not hold. Alleles located very close together tend to be transmitted as one unit to gametes, and their frequency cannot be predicted simply by the allele frequencies of each separate locus. Haplotypes consisting of particular allele pairs will occur at much greater frequency than expected

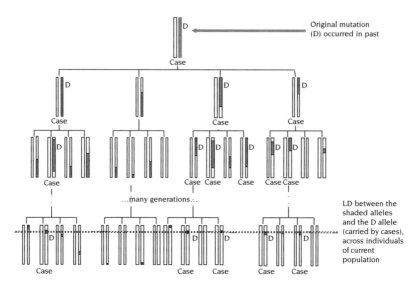

Figure 8.4. Linkage Disequilibrium (LD) over Generations

under linkage equilibrium when the loci are close together, and are therefore considered in linkage disequilibrium (LD). This creates correlation among alleles of separate loci across individuals. As shown in Figure 8.4, the "D" allele that is a risk factor for disease is correlated (in LD) with other alleles designated by the gray shading in the current population. Any marker located in the shaded region should show association with the disease, even if the "D" locus itself is not genotyped. This is a fundamental concept for using polymorphisms that are genetic "markers" as exposures for indirect tests in genetic epidemiology, as described below.

8.2.2.5 *Direct versus indirect association.* Based on the type of exposure examined, case-control studies of measured genotypes may be divided into two broad categories—direct and indirect association studies. For direct association studies, the genetic polymorphisms examined are the functional or causal SNPs in candidate genes, whereas indirect studies rely on genetic polymorphisms as "markers" of genomic regions. Therefore, in direct studies, the genetic exposure is directly measured, while for indirect studies, the genetic exposure is indirectly measured using markers as a proxy for exposure status (see Figure 8.5).

Direct studies test a very specific hypothesis that a causative SNP is associated with risk for the disease. An example of a direct association study is a case-control study of venous thrombosis conducted by Margaglione et al. (3). Two functional SNPs (G20210A of Prothrombin and

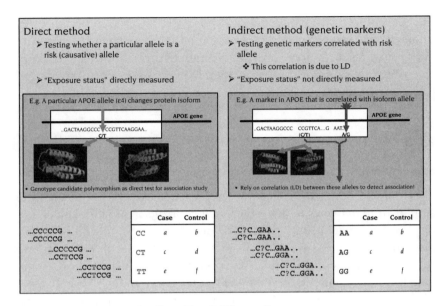

Figure 8.5. Association Studies—Two Different Concepts

the Factor V Leiden mutation) were studied in 281 cases with venous thrombosis (consecutive patients recruited from 2 thrombosis centers in southern Italy) and 850 healthy population-based controls. The odds ratio (OR) of venous thrombosis associated with carrying the A20210 allele in Prothrombin was 2.51 (95% CI: 1.29–4.22), and the OR of venous thrombosis associated with Factor V Leiden carriers was 3.24 (95% CI: 2.03–5.16).

On the other hand, indirect association studies aim to detect causative SNPs via their correlation with genetic markers. This is advantageous since the risk-conferring polymorphism or mutation may not be known; therefore, its location and genotyping assay are not available. Polymorphisms that are currently known in genes are used as genetic markers in hopes of capturing association between a marker and disease risk, due to the correlation between alleles of the marker, and alleles of the (unmeasured) risk polymorphism (see Figure 8.4). This assumed correlation between marker alleles and risk alleles is based on the assumption of LD between closely located loci. It is this property of LD that makes the use of genetic markers as proxy exposures possible for genetic epidemiology studies. Since indirect association studies do not directly assess the causative exposure, the magnitude of association between case-control status and the marker genotypes depends greatly on the LD structure that underlies these markers (e.g., SNPs). This is analogous to the concept of misclassification of exposure status in traditional epide-miology studies when proxy measures are used. Assessment of exposure via a proxy results in some misclassification of the true underlying expo-sure status thus diluting the association between case-control status and the proxy exposure measure.

8.3 CASE-CONTROL DESIGN

8.3.1 Description

Case-control designs for hypotheses related to genetic exposures are similar in many ways to any other case-control sampling in epidemiol-ogy. Cases are defined as having the disease of interest, while controls are those individuals from the same sampling frame who do not have the disease of interest. Controls may or may not be matched on partic-ular factors, depending on the potential for confounding. Several types of controls may be selected for genetic association studies with several selection strategies commonly in practice, including unrelated controls or unaffected twins or siblings (4). In most instances, the most desirable and suitable group of controls is a set of population-based controls, obtained as a random sample of individuals without disease selected from the source population of cases. This is especially practical for case-control studies that are nested within prospective cohort studies. One special consideration regarding controls for genetic studies is the poten-tial for confounding due to ethnicity/genetic background differences between cases and controls, which is discussed in more detail at the end of this section.

8.3.2 Methods of Analysis

8.3.2.1 *Frequency comparisons.* Association between a polymorphism and case-control status can be assessed by means of ORs and χ^2 tests. We will use SNPs as the assumed polymorphism type for the rest of this chapter. Furthermore, we will assume two alleles, A and a, for this SNP, with "a" being the at-risk allele. To test for genotypic effects of this biallelic SNP (A or a), a 3×2 contingency table is set up with two columns for case-control status and three rows for genotypes, as shown in Table 8.2. Using genotype (aa) as a reference group, the odds of cases having either the heterozygous genotype (Aa) or the homozy-gous at-risk genotype (AA) is compared to the odds of controls having one of those two genotypes. If the OR is not equal to 1, then an associa-tion between SNP and outcome exists. Alternatively, genotype groups

Table 8.2. Case-Control Study Of Single SNP

SNP Genotype	Controls	Cases	Odds Ratio
aa	a	b	1
Aa	c	d	$(d/b)/(c/a) = ad/bc$
AA	e	f	$(f/b)/(e/a) = af/be$

Table 8.3. Case-Control Study of Factor V Leiden Mutation and Venous Thrombosis

Factor V Leiden Mutation	Controls	Venous Thrombosis	OR (95% CI)
Noncarrier	807	230	1
Carrier	43	51	4.16 (2.70–6.14)

can be collapsed to test specific mode of inheritance of that SNP. For example, in the case-control of venous thrombosis by Margaglione et al. (3), the effect of Factor V Leiden mutation has previously been shown to act through dominant mode of inheritance, that is, the phenotype of individuals with one or two copies of the mutation was the same. Therefore, in the calculation of the OR for venous thrombosis, carriers of the mutation are compared to noncarriers, thus reducing the 2 × 3 table to a 2 × 2 table (Table 8.3).

8.3.2.2 *Regression models.* Case-control studies of genetic markers can be modeled using logistic regression, where the log odds of being a case is modeled as a function of the genotypes. Maximization techniques to esti-mate this regression parameter are available in most software packages, as are hypothesis testing options such as Wald tests or likelihood ratio tests. The logistic regression model expresses the relationship between a binary outcome (case-control status) and an exposure (genotype) in the following function:

$$\Pr(Y = 1 \mid X = Aa \, or \, AA) = \frac{1}{1 + e^{-(\beta_0 + \beta_1 X)}}$$

where $P(Y=1 \mid X = Aa \, or \, AA)$ denotes the probability (P) of the binary outcome (Y) for a given value of X (genotype = Aa or AA, assuming a dominant mode of inheritance). The interpretation of the exponentiated beta coefficient is the relative odds of being a case comparing those with either the Aa or AA genotypes to those with the aa genotype. If the OR is greater than 1, then cases are more likely to have either the Aa or AA genotypes. Logistic regressions allow for adjustment for potential confounders, assessment of potential mediating factors, and assessment of interactions with other genetic or environmental risk factors.

8.3.2.3 *Alleles versus genotypes.* The association between a SNP and case-control status may also examined on the allelic level. For example, Table 8.4 shows the relationship between the isoform polymorphism of the APOE gene and Alzheimer's disease at the allelic and genotype levels (5). In the allele situation, frequency of the at-risk allele is compared between cases and controls. Since the comparison is made on the allelic level, the total number of observations in a study is the number of chromosomes, that is, twice the number of people, and the allele frequency is defined as the number of at-risk alleles over the total number of alleles present. Allele frequencies are compared between cases and controls using the chi-squared test. Although allelic associations are more statistically powerful as the effective sample size is doubled, many epidemiologists are not in favor of this approach because other risk factors are measured on an individual, rather than chromosomal, level.

8.3.2.4 *Genetic models.* Although the example shown in Section 8.3.2.2 assumed a dominant mode of inheritance in the logistic regression modeling of the association between case-control status and genotype, different modes of inheritance can be modeled in the logistic framework, including codominant, additive, multiplicative, dominant, or recessive models. The most robust modeling makes no assumption about mode of inheritance, and simply considers risk for heterozygotes separately from risk to homozygotes for a risk allele. To achieve this codominant model, two variables are created: $X1 = 1$ if the genotype is heterozygote (e.g., Aa) and 0 otherwise, $X2 = 1$ if the genotype is homozygous (e.g., AA), and 0 otherwise, assuming the alternative homozygote (aa) is the

Table 8.4. APOE Genotype and Allele Frequencies by Alzheimer's Disease (AD) Status

	Genotypes					Alleles		
	$\varepsilon3/\varepsilon3$	$\varepsilon2/\varepsilon3$	$\varepsilon2/\varepsilon4$	$\varepsilon3/\varepsilon4$	$\varepsilon4/\varepsilon4$	$\varepsilon2$	$\varepsilon3$	$\varepsilon4$
AD*	53	11	10	95	21	21	212	147
($n = 190$)	27.9%	5.8%	5.3%	50.0%	11.1%	5.5%	55.8%	38.7%
Controls	86	13	2	28	3	15	213	36
(n = 132)	65.2%	9.8%	1.5%	21.2%	2.3%	5.7%	80.7%	13.6%
	$\chi^2 = 57.14$, df = 4, $P < 0.001$					$\chi^2 = 52.22$, df = 2, $P < 0.001$		

*Age of Onset $\geq$ 60 years

baseline. Typically the baseline is taken as the most common homozygous genotype, unless there is a reason to specify otherwise. Both variables are modeled in the logistic regression, and the exponentiated beta coefficient for X1 is the OR estimate for the outcome comparing Aa to aa while the exponentiated beta coefficient for X2 is the OR for the outcome comparing homozygous carriers (AA) to noncarriers (aa).

Although this codominant modeling is robust to mode of inheritance, it requires an additional degree of freedom. If an algebraic relationship can be established between heterozygote and homozygote risk, a more parsimonious model can be used. These include additive (where risk to AA is twice that of Aa), multiplicative (where risk to AA is the square of the risk to Aa), dominant (risk to AA is equal to risk for Aa), and recessive (only AA is at increased risk, and Aa risk is equal to baseline). These require only one variable in the logistic regression, with coded values corresponding to the model of interest. These are shown in Table 8.5. In practice, one may first consider the codominant model, and observe whether the X1 and X2 beta estimates and corresponding ORs fit one of these reduced models.

8.3.2.5. *Multiple loci.* When multiple SNPs are studied in a gene or in a region, each SNP can be independently tested for association with disease, or haplotypes may also be constructed for further analysis if the SNPs are in linkage disequilibrium with each other. There are several reasons to conduct multilocus haplotype analysis. First, because each new mutation is associated with a particular chromosomal background, haplotype-based analyses can detect unique chromosomal segments that may harbor the disease-causing allele. Second, a haplotype constructed from several SNPs provides increased informativity over single SNPs. Finally, biologically, combinations of alleles in a gene or a region may be

Table 8.5. Design Coding for Different Genetic Models

Genotype	Codominant		Additive*	Multiplicative*	Dominant	Recessive
	X1	X2	X	X	X	X
Aa	0	0	0	0	0	0
Aa	1	0	1	1	1	0
AA	0	1	2	2	1	1
Parameters estimated:	OR_{Aa}	OR_{AA}	OR_{Aa} $(OR_{AA} = 2*OR_{Aa})$	OR_{Aa} $(OR_{AA} = OR_{Aa}^2)$	OR_{A}-- $(OR_{AA} = OR_{Aa})$	OR_{AA} $(OR_{Aa} = OR_{aa} = 1)$

*Interpretation of model and parameters depends on scale. Multiplicative is assumed when employing this design coding in a logistic model.

functionally important so that a set of variants on a haplotype may be the causative "composite allele" rather than a particular allele of a SNP.

Analogous to genotype-based analysis, haplotype-based analyses compare frequencies of haplotypes between cases and controls. An association between disease and genetic variations is established if the distribution of haplotype frequencies differs between cases and controls. Unlike genotypes, which can be analyzed directly, haplotypes must first be constructed from multiple SNPs. Since human beings are diploids (containing one chromosome from each parent), haplotypes are typically established by genotyping family members to infer parental chromosomes. This becomes impractical and expensive for diseases that are late-onset and for studies that did not recruit multi-generational families. Therefore, alternative methods were developed to establish haplotypes in case-control studies of unrelated individuals. These methods include laboratory-based techniques which amplify long chromosomal segments (long-range PCR) and statistical methods which estimate haplotype frequencies based on genotypes. A number of different methods for estimating haplotypes in unrelated individuals, such as the Expectation-Maximization algorithm (6) or Bayesian methods (7), exist, but the details of these methods are beyond the scope of this chapter.

8.3.3 Confounding due to Ancestry in Case-Control Studies of Genetic Risk Factors (Sometimes Called Population Stratification)

As previously mentioned, a noncausal association between a SNP and case-control status may exist simply because cases and controls have different allele frequencies due to differences in genetic background. A classic example of confounding by genetic ancestry was demonstrated by Knowler et al. in a study of HLA haplotypes and type 2 diabetes in Pima Indians (8). Epidemiologic studies have consistently shown higher prevalence and incidence of type 2 diabetes in Pima Indians compared to U.S. whites. In this study, the Gm3;5,13,14 haplotype was strongly associated with a lower prevalence of type 2 diabetes (prevalence ratio = 0.27, 95% CI: 0.18–0.40) in a group of Pima Indians. However, after furthermore examination, Knowler et al. showed that this haplotype is simply an index for white admixture. The frequency of this particular haplotype is lower in whites than in Pima Indians; therefore, Pima Indians with more white admixture were more likely to have the Gm3;5,13,14 haplotype than those who were full-heritage Pima Indians. Consequently, when all individuals were analyzed without taking degree of admixture into consideration, the Gm3;5,13,14 was associated with lower prevalence of type 2 diabetes. When the analysis was stratified by degree of admixture, no association between the

Gm3;5,13,14 haplotype and type 2 diabetes was observed in either the full-heritage Pima-Indian group or the groups with varying degrees of white admixture.

A few solutions during the design phase of a study exist for the problem of population stratification. One solution is to collect information on ethnicity and then to either select controls that are matched to the cases on ethnicity or perform stratified analysis according to ethnicity. However, this is not a perfect solution because it is almost impossible to match for all differences in genetic background between cases and controls. Furthermore, self-reported ethnicity may reflect more strongly heterogeneity in cultural differences between population subgroups than heterogeneity in genetic backgrounds. Another solution to this problem is to use family members as controls, which is one of the best ways to match on genetic backgrounds but may often be impractical and inefficient. One such control is an unaffected sibling (discordant sib pair design) because these individuals are more likely to be in the age range as the cases (or matched by age in the case of twins). One potential problem with sibling controls is that younger siblings may not have had time to develop disease; therefore, older siblings are generally preferred as the discordant sib control. Another popular family-based design is the parent-case trio, using the transmission-disequilibrium test (TDT), which is discussed in Section 8.4.

If it is not possible to select family-based controls who would match cases with respect to genetic background, one can assess the problem of population stratification between cases and unrelated controls by collecting genotype data from anonymous markers throughout the genome. The basic principle is that anonymous markers throughout the genome should be an indicator of the diversity of genetic background amongst individuals as long as these markers are not associated with the outcome (9). This, in essence, utilizes molecular technology, rather than self-report of ancestry, to characterize an individual's genetic background. If population stratification is detected, several methods have been proposed to use these markers in the analysis phase. These include rescaling the chi-squared statistic in the association test or using the anonymous markers to divide cases and controls into subgroups with more genetic homogeneity (10,11).

8.4 CASE-PARENT TRIO DESIGN

8.4.1 Description

A second method for assessing genes as risk factors for disease is to sample affected individuals (cases), and their parents. In this setting, parental genotypes are used as controls. This is based on Mendel's law that parental alleles are transmitted to each child with equal chance (50:50 probability). Of the two parental alleles for any marker, one is the allele that was transmitted to the affected child, while the other was not transmitted. The transmitted allele, carried by the affected offspring, is the "case" allele, while the nontransmitted parent allele is the "control" allele. According to Mendel's law, either could have been transmitted to the case with equal probability. Therefore, across parents with the same two alleles, 50% of the children should have received one kind of allele, and 50% the other kind (see Figure 8.6). This is the null hypothesis of the TDT, which treats each allele carried by an affected offspring as a "case allele" or "transmitted allele," and each nontransmitted parent allele as a "control" allele, in a matched parent-case pair setting. Because the case-parent trio design samples only cases, there will be greater than 50% transmission of risk alleles (or alleles in LD with risk alleles) among the sampled parent-affected child pairs, since the risk allele would be oversampled from the general population by sampling only cases (see Figure 8.6). The TDT therefore tests for over-transmission of a particular allele as evidence of association between that locus and disease status. The particular statistical implementations for the case-parent design are described in this section.

8.4.2 *Methods of Analysis for the Case-Parent Trio Design*

8.4.2.1 *McNemar's test.* The original transmission-disequilibrium test (TDT) compares alleles transmitted to cases with parental alleles not transmitted to cases, by setting up a table of matched transmitted/

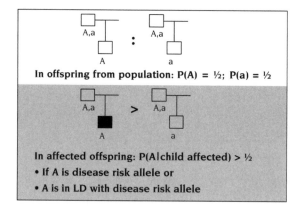

Figure 8.6. Transmission from Parent to Offspring under Mendel's Law, and When Sampling Cases Only

nontransmitted alleles for each parent-case pair. Figure 8.7 shows how some example trios would contribute to a matched transmission table, with each trio contributing 2 matched pair observations. Under the null hypothesis of 50:50 transmission of parental alleles to offspring, the top right and bottom left "discordant" cells should have equal counts, or their ratio of counts should equal 1. In other words, among heterozygous parents, which allele is "transmitted" should be either version with equal frequency. Any departure from an expected ratio of 1, is evidence for over- or under-transmission of a particular allele to affected offspring. These "off-diagonal" counts are then used in a McNemar's test to assess association between a particular allele and case status. The OR for this association can also be estimated as b/c. As an example, Ogura et al. (12) examined a single base pair insertion in the NOD2 gene (3020insC) on chromosome 16 among Crohn's Disease cases and their parents, and found among 56 heterozygous parents, 39 transmitted the insertion to their affected child, and 17 did not ($\chi^2 = 8.64$, $P = 0.0046$, OR $= 2.29$).

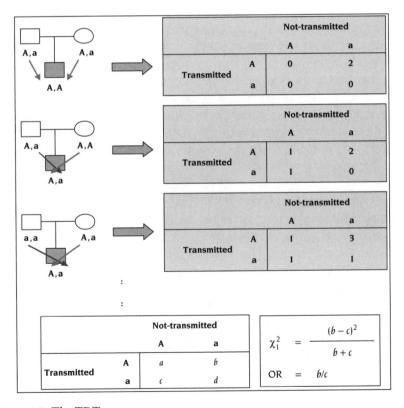

Figure 8.7. The TDT

8.4.2.2 *Regression modeling.* The original TDT can also be modeled using conditional logistic regression, where the log odds of being a transmitted allele, versus a nontransmitted allele, given each parent-offspring pair, is modeled as a function of the particular allele. Maximization techniques to estimate this regression parameter are available in most software packages, as are hypothesis testing options such as Wald tests or likelihood ratio tests.

$$\ln\left(\frac{P(transmitted \mid X, parent)}{1 - P(transmitted \mid X, parent)}\right) = \alpha + \beta X_=$$

For example, Maestri et al. (13) used this approach to estimate the effect of alleles in TGFB3 on risk for oral clefts among 160 case-parent trios. Using this approach, a particular allele of the STR D14S61 in that gene (coded as allele 6) had a higher odds of being a case allele than a nontransmitted parental allele (OR = 1.84). The traditional TDT approach showed this allele was transmitted from heterozygous parents to cleft cases 46 times, versus 26 times that it was not transmitted from a heterozygous parent to an affected child in the study (OR = 48/26 = 1.84), which is consitent with the conditional logistic estimate. The authors then use the flexibility of this framework to incorporate additional variables that may contribute to genetic heterogeneity. By including an interaction term for the product of allele 6 status and whether the mother smoked during pregnancy, they were able to show increased risk for the risk allele among smoking mothers (OR = 5.33) versus nonsmoking mothers (OR = 1.54), and to test for this interaction via likelihood ratio tests.

8.4.2.3 *Allelic versus Genotypic TDT.* The original TDT using a McNemar's matched chi-squared test, or using the conditional logistic regression approach above consider transmission of alleles, and are therefore tests of 2N alleles, rather than N genotypes. This is analogous to considering the case-control tests of association described in the previous section at either the allelic (2N), or genotypic (N) levels. One can recast the case-parent trio information as a test of genotypes, by considering each trio as a single matched set. In this scenario, there are four possible offspring genotypes for each set of parents, according to Mendelian laws. Under the null hypothesis of no association, any offspring has a 25% chance of getting one of these four possible genotypes. Across families sampled on case status, if any one genotype occurs much more than 25% of the time, this is evidence against the null, in favor of association between

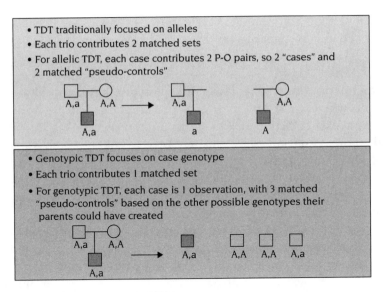

Figure 8.8. Allelic vs Genotypic TDT

that genotype and risk for the disease. This can be modeled as a 1:3 matched set in a conditional logistic framework, with the affected offspring's genotype considered a "case" and the other three possible genotypes, given the parents, as "pseudosibling controls" (see Figure 8.8).

8.4.2.4 *Genetic models.* Casting the TDT in genotype units, rather than alleles, has the advantage of considering the appropriate number of observations (N cases, or N matched sets, versus 2N matched pairs). In addition, it allows appropriate modeling of genetic risk, as discussed for case-control studies in Section 8.3.2.4, and in Table 8.4. For example, the most robust modeling would be to consider heterozygote and homozygote carriers of a risk allele separately, without assuming a mathematical relationship between them.

$$\ln\left[\frac{P(Transmitted \mid I, parents)}{1 - P(Transmitted \mid I, parents)}\right] = \alpha + \beta_1 I_{Aa} + \beta_2 I_{AA}$$

This requires two regression parameters, but makes no assumptions about the underlying genetic model. In contrast, if a genetic model is known, or can be safely assumed, this could be reduced to one parameter, under a particular genetic model scenario (see Table 8.4).

The conditional logistic framework has the advantage of allowing additional terms for interactions between genes, or between genes and environments. This can also be accomplished through log-linear regression modeling, as suggested by Umbach and Weinberg (14).

8.4.2.5 *Multiple loci.* As discussed in Section 8.3.2.5, analysis of multiple SNPs simultaneously, in the form of haplotypes, has many advantages, and can increase the power to detect associations when a haplotype pattern acts as a better marker of an underlying risk allele than any single polymorphism. Unfortunately, even though families provide more phase information than unrelated individuals, phase often still cannot be resolved unambiguously within a family; several haplotype phases may be consistent with the multiple genotypes observed. This requires a phase estimation step using EM or Bayesian methods as mentioned in Section 8.3.2.4, which are outside the scope of this chapter. However, assuming phase can be established for each trio, one can carry out an allelic of genotypic TDT by treating a multilocus haplotype as an "allele" of pair of haplotypes as a "genotype" in the TDT methods described above. To perform the traditional allelic TDT, one would tally which haplotype was transmitted to an affected offspring among a set of (haplotype) heterozygous parents. For example, Hugot et al. (15) genotyped 8 SNPs in the NOD2 gene on chromosome 16 among 235 Crohn's Disease cases and their parents, then created 6-SNP haplotypes based on these genotypes. Table 8.6 shows the tally of transmitted to nontransmitted haplotypes, considering each haplotype as the target "risk" haplotype for analysis. Haplotype 21111122 shows the strongest evidence for excess transmission among these Crohn's Disease trios, with two other haplotypes, sharing the first four SNP alleles in common, also showing evidence for association.

Table 8.6. Haplotype TDT Analyses from Hugot et al. (15) for common haplotypes based on 8 SNPs in NOD2

Haplotype								Trans	Not Trans	P Value
2	1	1	1	2	1	2	1	82	48	0.001
2	1	1	1	1	2	2	1	38	13	0.0005
2	1	1	1	1	1	2	2	83	22	0.0000002
1	2	2	2	1	1	1	1	116	141	NS*
1	2	2	1	1	1	1	1	9	19	NS
1	2	2	1	1	1	2	1	94	116	NS
2	2	2	1	1	1	2	1	20	16	NS
2	1	1	1	1	1	2		701	78	NS

*NS = not significant.

8.4.3 Issues to Be Considered

Whether considering case-parent matched pairs of alleles, or case-pseudosibling matched sets of genotypes, one important aspect of the case-parent trio design is the need for heterozygous parents. Otherwise, only equivocal information is provided. Therefore, the power of any case-parent trio design depends on the number of heterozygous parents one can expect for a particular polymorphism to be genotyped. As allele frequencies become more rare, the probability of heterozygote parents becomes more rare, and the number of trios needed to obtain informative families increases. However, this design has maintained popularity, due to several advantages. First, this genetically matched design avoids confounding due to ancestry by specifically matching controls on ancestry (other parent alleles). Second, this design allows for questions of parent-of-origin effects, such as imprinting, where risk for disease in the child depends on which parent gave a particular allele to that child. This type of effect is impossible to glean if parent genotypes are not collected.

8.5 CASE-ONLY DESIGNS

The case-only design has been proposed to be a more efficient design, both in terms of statistical power and data collection, for detecting gene-by-environment (G × E) interactions than traditional case-control designs (16). In this design, only cases are sampled from the general case population. This design can be related to the completed case-control framework as shown in Table 8.2. In the case-only design, a multiplicative interactive effect is modeled and estimated as an OR. The null hypothesis is that the OR for the outcome in those with both the gene and the environmental risk factors (OR_{GE}) will be equal to the product of ORs for each factor alone: that is, $OR_{GE} = OR_G \times OR_E$. Departure of the ratio of OR_{GE} to the product of OR_G and OR_E from 1 indicates the presence of multiplicative interaction (OR_{MI}). With this multiplicative framework, it has been shown that under the assumption of rare disease and independence between the genetic and the environmental factors in the population, the multiplicative interactive model represented in Table 8.7 can be simplified to $OR_{MI} = ag/ce$ (a represents the number of cases with both G and E factors, g represents number of cases with neither G nor E factor, c represents the number of cases with only the G factor, and e represents the number of cases with only the E factor), which is a function of the joint frequencies of genetic factor and environmental factors among cases. Thus, cases alone can be used to estimate interactions. The case-only design has been shown to be more efficient for

Table 8.7. Case-Only Design

G	E	Case	Control	Effect Estimator
+	+	a	b	$OR_{GE} = ah/bg$
+	–	c	d	$OR_G = ch/dg$
–	+	e	f	$OR_E = eh/fg$
–	–	g	h	–
				$OR_{MI} = OR_{GE}/(OR_G * OR_E)$

detecting $G \times E$ interaction than case-control studies, given the smaller variance based on four cells of individuals instead of eight cells of individuals in the complete case-control design.

8.6 SUMMARY AND GENERAL ISSUES FOR CASE-BASED GENETIC EPIDEMIOLOGY STUDIES

Genetic epidemiology is a field of science that focuses on the role of genetic factors and their interaction with environmental factors in the occurrence of disease in human populations (17). In this chapter, we introduced the field of genetic epidemiology in general, presenting the central paradigm (Figure 8.1) of first establishing familial aggregation and heritability, then searching for genetic risk factors through linkage or association studies. We then focused on the unique aspects of considering genes as risk factors in an epidemiological study, and specifically on the designs and analysis strategies within this paradigm that use case sampling approaches to evaluate the influence of genes on disease risk.

In Section 8.2.1, we showed how the classic case-control design can be used to assess familial aggregation of disease by simply using family history information (unmeasured genotypes). However, results from familial aggregation studies must be interpreted with caution as family members may also share environmental risk factors. In Section 8.3, we showed the use of the case-control design to examine associations between genetic markers (measured genotypes) and disease, in 8.4 we gave examples for use of the case-parent trio design, and finally in 8.5, we highlighted the potential utility and pitfalls of case-only designs. In these studies, genetic markers are treated as "exposure" variables, and association between disease and a marker is established when the odds ratio estimate departs from 1. Traditional guidelines regarding selection of representative cases and comparable controls, discussed elsewhere in this book, are equally applicable to case-control studies of genetic risk factors. In addition, extra attention must be paid to ensure that cases and controls are comparable with respect to their genetic background so that spurious associations as a result of confounding due to genetic ancestry are not reported. This has been one of the main advantages to the case-parent trio design.

The goal of this chapter is to introduce the common case-based genetic epidemiology designs, and the direct and indirect tests applied in these designs, to provide a foundation for understanding reports of genetic epidemiology studies. Table 8.8 summarizes some possible interpretations of positive and negative findings in genetic association studies, in the context of what has been presented in this chapter. A positive result (OR estimate significantly different than 1) may reflect a true causal relationship between the alleles measured and disease. However, the measured genotype may also reflect a marker that is in LD with a causal variant. The power to detect this association will depend on the magnitude of correlation (e.g., r^2) between that genotype and the underlying disease risk allele. However, a positive result could also occur due to confounding as a result of population stratification, or some other confounder, or simply due to sampling error. Similarly, several reasons can explain a lack of association, including lack of statistical power, or sampling error. Specifically, one may lack power due to poor coverage of the gene of interest, such that no marker genotyped for the study was actually in high LD with the underlying causal variant. Past candidate gene studies were often flawed in this way, studying only one or two polymorphisms per gene, greatly reducing the chance of detecting an association with parts of the gene not correlated to those markers.

Lastly, other case-based designs, such as the case-parent trio and the case-only, offer unique advantages for addressing specific questions. The case-parent trio avoids confounding by population stratification by

Table 8.8. Interpretation Of Positive And Negative Association Studies

A positive association can mean:
- The targeted allele is causal
- The targeted allele is in LD with a causal allele
- There is confounding due to population stratification
- There is confounding or bias for some other reason
- Type I error

A negative finding can mean:
- The gene or region under study is not associated with disease risk
- The targeted allele is not in LD with the causal allele
- Appropriate stratification or other accommodation of heterogeneity was not identified
- Type II error (not enough power)

using parental genotypes as the matched genetic controls in the analysis; however, potential difficulties in recruitment of parents for diseases with older age of onset may be problematic. The case-only design has been shown to be more statistically efficient for identification of gene-by-environment interactions; however, the assumption of independence between gene and environment in the control population must be met for this design to be valid.

In summary, several case-based designs are useful for studying genetic risk factors in the population. Although genetic case-control studies can not establish causality of genetic variations, they are efficient and can answer many questions regarding the role of genetic variations and disease risk in the population when they are well designed. The identification of causal genetic variants and their interactions with other genes and the environment is the ultimate goal of genetic epidemiology, and often one must take the associations detected via the work described in this chapter into the laboratory, to understand the functional role of any detected risk variants.

REFERENCES

1. Pankow JS, Folsom AR, Province MA,.et al. Family history of coronary heart disease and hemostatic variables in middle-aged adults. *Thrombosis and Haemostasis.* 1997;77(1):87-93.
2. Risch N. The genetic epidemiology of cancer: interpreting family and twin studies and their implications for molecular genetic approaches. *Cancer Epidemiol.Biomarkers Prev.* 2001;10(7):733-741.
3. Margaglione M, Brancaccio V, Giuliani N, et al. Increased risk for venous thrombosis in carriers of the prothrombin G-->A20210 gene variant. *Ann Intern Med.* 1998;129(2):89-93.
4. Witte JS, Gauderman WJ, Thomas DC. Asymptotic bias and efficiency in case-control studies of candidate genes and gene–environment interactions: Basic family designs. *Am J Epidemiol.* 1999;149 (8):693-705.
5. Mullan M, Scibelli P, Duara R, et al. Familial and population-based studies of apolipoprotein E and Alzheimer's disease. *Ann N Y Acad Sci.* 1996; 802:16-26.
6. Fallin D, Schork NJ. Accuracy of haplotype frequency estimation for biallelic loci, via the expectation-maximization algorithm for unphased diploid genotype data. *Am J Hum Genet.* 2000;67(4):947-959.
7. Stephens M, Smith NJ, Donnelly P. A new statistical method for haplotype reconstruction from population data. *Am J Hum Genet.* 2001;68(4):978-989.
8. Knowler WC, Williams RC, Pettitt DJ, Steinberg AG. Gm3;5,13,14 and type 2 diabetes mellitus: an association in American Indians with genetic admixture. *Am J Hum Genet.* 1988;43(4):520-526.
9. Pritchard JK, Rosenberg NA. Use of unlinked genetic markers to detect population stratification in association studies. *Am J Hum Genet.* 1999;65(1):220-228.

10. Pritchard JK, Stephens M, Donnelly P. Inference of population structure using multilocus genotype data. *Genetics*. 2000;155(2):945-959.
11. Devlin B, Roeder K. Genomic controls for association studies. *Biometrics*. 1999;55:997-1004.
12. Ogura Y, Bonen DK, Inohara N, et al. A frameshift mutation in NOD2 associated with susceptibility to Crohn's disease. *Nature*. 2001;411(6837):603-606.
13. Maestri NE, Beaty TH, Hetmanski J, et al. Application of transmission-disequilibrium tests to nonsyndromic oral clefts: including candidate genes and environmental exposures in the models. *Am J Med Genet*. 1997;73(3):337-344.
14. Umbach DH, Weinberg CR. The use of case-parent triads to study joint meets of genotype and exposure. *Am J Hum Genet*. 2000;66(1):251-261.
15. Hugot JP, Chamaillard M, Zouali H, et al. Association of NOD2 leucine-rich repeat variants with susceptibility to Crohn's disease.*Nature*. 2001; 411(6837):599-603.
16. Khoury MJ, Flanders WD. Nontraditional epidemiologic approaches in the analysis of gene–environment interaction: case-control studies with no controls! *Am.J.Epidemiol*. 1996;144(3):207-213.
17. Khoury MJ, Beaty TH, Cohen B. *Fundamentals of Genetic Epidemiology*. New York: Oxford University Press; 1993.

9

APPLICATIONS: EVALUATION

Haroutune K. Armenian

OUTLINE

This chapter aims to

1. list various approaches to evaluation and describe situations where one needs to have alternatives for randomized trials in assessing interventions;
2. identify circumstances that will benefit from the use of the case-control method as an approach for evaluation; and
3. present the example of the case-control method to evaluate vaccination programs.

9.1 EVALUATING HEALTH SERVICES

9.1.1 Overview

The evaluation of various activities and interventions in health services requires a data-information base that responds to a number of relevant questions. Epidemiology provides the appropriate methodology to generate responses to these questions. From surveillance data and descriptive surveys to observational analytic studies and randomized experimental trials, all epidemiologic methods can be used as tools for evaluation.

As presented in Table 9.1, a number of general and specific questions may serve as the basis for evaluative research. These include general questions regarding an appropriate community diagnosis of health problems, to more specific questions about the efficacy of various treatment modalities.

Essentially, evaluation provides the data for decision making at a number of levels for health services and for health care (1). Such decisions can be *political*—within the domain of the political process—and *managerial*—made by the health professionals at an operational level. Some of the political decisions include *budget and resource allocation*, defining the *jurisdiction of agencies*, selecting *political appointees* to key positions, and setting health care *legislation*.

9.1.2 Questions for Evaluation

Decisions made at the *operational and management* level include those concerning patient care or the *efficacy* of therapies, the *effectiveness* of

Table 9.1. Questions for Evaluation

What are the health problems faced?

To make a *community* diagnosis problems need to be defined as to their
• nature;
• magnitude;
• severity;
• distribution;
• trends.

What is being done to resolve these health problems?
We need to assess what are some of the *structures* developed in the community to deal with these problems as well as the health-care *processes* that are put to use to deal with these problems.

Are the problems being resolved and innovations improving matters?
Measuring changes in *outcomes* is the most direct way of demonstrating the *effectiveness* of our interventions

---

interventions in the community, the *quality* of the health services, and the *planning and programming* for services.

Evaluative studies in epidemiology have a primary focus on generating information about *efficacy* or the ability of an intervention to achieve targeted outcomes *under ideal conditions,-* such as in a controlled trial—and also about *effectiveness* or the ability of an intervention or program to achieve desired results in a *community-based ongoing environment* of utilization. Epidemiologists may also be engaged in assessing *efficiency* or the intensity of *use of resources* to achieve certain objectives.

To generate the appropriate database for these decisions in health services, one may use a number of approaches. Some of the simplest of these approaches include basic *clinical impressions* (this treatment works very well in my experience), some individual *case reports* that support a claim of efficacy, or similarly, a *series of cases* where the evaluator has observed some response or lack of it.

The data collection for such observations is not limited to the clinical set up and may involve a *survey* in the community. All these approaches are in the framework of *uncontrolled* evaluative research. For example, in a study of the 1993 epidemic of pertussis in Cincinnati, Christie et al. (2) reviewed 255 cases of the disease and reported that over 74% of these cases were appropriately immunized with pertussis vaccine previously. They concluded from a study of this case series that the existing pertussis v23ccine "failed to give full protection against the disease."

As stated in Chapter 1, the presence of a comparison group strengthens the argument about the observed associations. Similarly, in evaluation, we need the comparison group for appropriate inferences. *Comparative* evaluation studies include *before–after* studies involving the comparison of a community or an institution before and after the implementation of a program or specific interventions. For example, one may study the incidence of advanced cervical cancer and its mortality in a community before and after the introduction of a massive pap smear cervical cancer-screening program or more recently following the introduction of the human Papillomavirus vaccine. One difficulty with such an evaluation is that other concurrent changes in the community may affect the results of the study in addition to the intervention.

Better-organized evaluation of services and interventions can be conducted using analytic designs in epidemiology. These include *cohort* studies in a population or community where there has been some use of the treatment or intervention and the *case-control* method, the topical area to be covered by this chapter.

The use of observational methods to assess therapies and interventions has been established at the core of a number of programs involved in outcomes research whereby currently used therapies are assessed for effectiveness and efficacy. Observational methods make it possible for massive amounts of recorded data to be used for the evaluation of interventions and practice patterns (3). With all these designs, one needs to assume the principle that, at baseline, the comparison groups are at equal risk of developing the outcome or disorder regardless of exposure to the intervention (4).

Observational controlled studies such as the case-control and cohort studies are able to primarily measure effectiveness because they assess the impact of an intervention under natural or routine circumstances. Also, most of the experimental or controlled trials are conducted under circumstances that are close to ideal and aim primarily at measuring efficacy. The difference between the controlled experimental trial and the observational study is more than the unbiased allocation and control of the treatment or intervention between the study groups. Observational studies are affected by differentials in methods of assessment of diagnosis and allotment of treatment modalities, as well as patient adherence to treatment, socioeconomic influences, and access to care (5). These are some of the factors where differentials between groups make it difficult to obtain a valid assessment of efficacy through an observational study.

A number of *problems arise with using observational studies* to evaluate therapies and interventions. These include *selection* biases, since allocation of therapy or interventions to individuals in the general population is never at random and may be influenced by a variety of factors that can act as confounders. A well-established bias under these circumstances is *confounding by indication* (6).

People are selected to receive a treatment or a vaccine on the basis of an assessment that includes severity of the condition, the potential risk of the individual to develop certain complications, or end points. Thus, the decision on exposure (treatment) is very much dependent on the potential of the individual for developing the outcome. In an observational study we need to assess the impact of selection on the basis of indication by inquiring about such selection factors in both cases and controls. Similarly, there may be a process of self-selection of individuals toward one or another treatment options based on a personal assessment or appreciation of risk for outcome.

It is also possible that persons receiving a particular treatment or those exposed to a certain intervention may be more closely monitored for the outcome of disease than others not receiving such an intervention. This may result in a *detection bias*, which can be measured if the appropriate information is collected about the intensity of diagnostic surveillance, and if measures of such intensity of surveillance are included in our comparisons or in our analysis.

The gold standard for evaluation research in epidemiology is the *controlled experimental or clinical trial*, where the investigator is able to *control the allocation* of the treatment to the various study groups. A number of variants of the controlled clinical trial are described in numerous texts on the subject. Such a trial involves designating a test and control treatment or intervention, developing a protocol for treatment administration and data collection, enrolling suitable patients, collecting data about baseline measures to monitor subsequent changes in the study subjects, assigning the treatments or intervention via some means that is free of selection and other biases, and following up the study subjects for specified outcomes and potential adverse effects of the treatment. Two assumptions underlie the use of clinical trials, particularly randomized trials. First, randomization prevents bias by establishing an allocation system of the intervention to be evaluated independently from the risk for the outcomes, and second, randomization is necessary for the valid interpretation of statistical significance, as stated by R.A. Fisher (7).

However, there are a number of problems that one needs to recognize prior to implementing such a trial. One needs to consider that most clinical trials require a large budget and other important technical and structural *resources*, that there are a number of *ethical constraints* that may not allow us to embark on a particular trial, and that sometimes the outcomes to be observed may have a very *long period of latency* and it may be decades before one is able to make some inferences about efficacy and effectiveness. Some clinical trials are developed under ideal experimental circumstances and it may be difficult to judge whether the observed findings are applicable in real-life situations. Thus, the conditions under which a controlled trial is conducted may be very different from using the same intervention routinely by the health services. For example, the investigator will make sure that a vaccine is properly stored and administered in a controlled trial while the conditions of storage and administration may not be ideal in a health center where the vaccine is given as part of routine health care (8,9).

There may be circumstances whereby the efficacy of a certain intervention is properly established by a controlled trial but changes in the process of administration, and differences in population characteristics may dictate a review of the assessment of the intervention's efficacy under such circumstances. It may be difficult for the investigator to ethically justify a new clinical trial in this situation.

When the intervention has already been implemented for a purpose other than our primary concern, we may decide not to conduct a controlled trial and start with an observational study to assess effectiveness for this second outcome. For example, it has been hypothesized that nonsteroidal anti-inflammatory drugs (NSAIDs) may be protective for colon cancer that has an induction time of several decades. Embarking on a clinical trial to test these drugs as a preventive measure for colon cancer may be difficult to justify both in terms of cost and of the difficulty of setting up such a study over a number of decades. As millions of people are users of these NSAIDs for arthritis and other inflammatory conditions, we need first to conduct a number of observational studies in the general population to test the effectiveness of these drugs in preventing cancer of the colon. Working on a similar hypothesis, Sivak-Sears et al. (10) conducted a case-control study of a highly malignant brain tumor, glioblastoma multiforme (GBM), and the potential protective effect of NSAIDs on these tumors. They compared 236 cases of GBM and 401 population-based controls, frequency matched on age, gender, and ethnicity from the San Francisco area. Cases reported less use of at least 600 pills of all types of NSAIDs combined during the 10-year prediagnostic period than did the controls (OR = 0.53, 95% CI: 0.3, 0.8). The ORs for the individual NSAIDs analyzed separately were very similar to the combined results.

In addition to those described above a number of areas are not suitable or practical to be tested through controlled experimental trials. These include the investigation of treatment toxicities, the detection of and estimation of rare outcomes, and assessment of lifelong effects.

As stated by Hellman and Hellman (11), "It is fallacious to suggest that only the randomized clinical trial can provide valid information or that all information acquired by this technique is valid. Such experimental methods are intended to reduce error and bias and therefore reduce the uncertainty of the result. Uncertainty cannot be eliminated, however."

9.2 EVALUATION USING THE CASE-CONTROL APPROACH

9.2.1 Overview

Over the past two decades a number of techniques have been used to improve the inferences made from observational evaluative studies. These include efforts at accounting or measuring the effect of various potential biases and confounders; examples include assessing intensity of diagnostic monitoring or ascertaining indices of severity of illness in the study groups.

As the case-control studies of the evaluation of various interventions are conducted in the community during "normal" conditions of use, the estimates obtained from these studies are more akin to effectiveness studies than efficacy studies. In the latter type of studies, through randomization or other approaches, one is able to establish a high level of comparability between those getting the intervention and those who are not. Thus, we end up in these trials with the highest level of comparability as to known but also unknown confounders. In an observational case-control study, although one may not have such ideal conditions as to the control of confounders as in a randomized trial, one may test for comparability of the two groups of exposure in the cases and controls as to all the known confounders. Within such a case-control study, a high level of comparability on known confounders of people exposed to the intervention and those who are not exposed makes our ascertainment of the effect of the intervention closer to an efficacy study than an effectiveness study.

There are a number of advantages for using the case-control method for the evaluation of interventions. The *efficiency* of the method in addressing the question with *fewer study* subjects, in a *shorter time frame* and with *less cost* can present a major advantage. Compared to controlled trials, and as an observational study, the method has *fewer ethical constraints* and no stopping rules. The case-control method provides *estimates of effect that are more realistic* than in an experimentally selected environment.

As a design the case-control method allows the assessment of more than one intervention, therapy, or regimen. Although a randomized trial may be able to incorporate two to four different arms of intervention, the case-control study may be able to compare all of the available interventions in the community, as well as investigate potential interactions between them. In a case-control study one may be able to assess the effect of changes in doses and other effects of differences of patterns of use of the therapy or intervention. Because in a case-control study one is able to have the largest number of people at risk of the outcome, the study may have more power to examine the effect of multiple therapies and their interactions.

In applying the case-control method to evaluation, however, there are a number of concerns, including lack of randomness in selecting study subjects and their exposure to the interventions under consideration, and the knowledge that the study will provide an assessment of effectiveness rather than efficacy in almost all situations.

One of the problems with using the case-control method in evaluation is that one is limited to assess the effect of the intervention(s) on one outcome that defines the case status. In a number of studies we may be interested in assessing the effect of the treatment on more than one outcome. For example, we may be interested in the side effects of the treatment as well as survival with the condition. Thus, we may need to set up two case-control studies, one with cases defined as people who died from the disease and a second study where the cases are those who developed the side effects of the therapy.

Other problems with case-control studies of evaluation include potential *information biases*. We may be able to get better treatment information from those who have developed some complications or who were not very successful with the treatment than from those who do not have the outcome. Also, important details about exposure to therapy or intervention such as frequency, dose, and skipping patterns may be missed in the controls when compared to the cases.

9.2.2 Examples

Over the past few decades, the case-control method has been used for evaluating a large number of interventions and therapies (12), and a number of examples follow.

9.2.2.1 *Effectiveness of drugs.* Controversy has existed for a number of decades about the effectiveness of anticoagulants in preventing hospital mortality in the post myocardial period. Two independent case-control studies by Tonascia et al. (13) and by Modan et al. (14) showed a significant reduction in short-term hospital mortality for patients receiving anticoagulants. Nonsteroidal anti-inflammatory drugs (NSAIDs) may help prevent breast cancer. Kirsh et al. (15) examined the association between regular NSAID use and the risk of breast cancer in 3,125 cases of breast cancer and an age-matched, random sample of 3,062 controls. NSAID use was associated with reduced breast cancer risk (OR = 0.76, 95% CI: 0.66, 0.88). The magnitude of this inverse association was similar for women with or without arthritis and within the different smoking strata.

9.2.2.2 *Adverse drug reactions.* One of the important questions that an assessment of a new drug or intervention would need to answer is the risk of adverse reactions in people who are taking the new drug. Classic examples of case-control studies of adverse reactions are those conducted in the 1970s and 1980s in the context of the Boston Collaborative Drug Surveillance Program (16). During the same period, a number of case-control studies focused on adverse reactions, such as peripheral thromboembolic disease following the use of estrogens and oral contraceptives. The advantage of the case-control method in the evaluation of adverse drug effects is that we are able to study long-term effects of drugs at times over many decades. Cook et al. (17) evaluated whether a mother's use of specific medications during pregnancy and lactation was involved in the development of neuroblastoma in the offspring. They compared 504 incident cases of neuroblastoma and age-matched controls selected from the same community by random digit dialing as to exposures to medications. Mothers of cases were more likely to report intake of opioid agonists and codeine than control mothers.

9.2.2.3 *Vaccines.* The evaluation of the effectiveness and possibly the efficacy of vaccines using the case-control method will be discussed later in this chapter.

9.2.2.4 *Screening programs.* Chapter 10 will present some of the unusual features of the case-control method as used extensively in the assessment of screening programs.

9.2.2.5 *Quality of care.* Most quality assurance programs are limited to an evaluation based on a comparison between the type of care provided to a series of cases and some external standard established by leaders of the profession. The focus of a case-control study of quality of care will be on outcomes, and some internal comparisons will be used. Thus cases of adverse outcome in a certain group of patients will be compared with controls without that adverse outcome, but with the same basic condition. The two groups will be compared as to their differences in medical care.

9.2.2.6 *Nutrition.* Similarly, a group with a certain diagnosis can be compared to a group of controls without such diagnosis as to differences in nutritional patterns.

9.2.2.7 *Public health programs.* The government of Lesotho and UNICEF had embarked on a program of building household latrines in villages to prevent diarrheal disease, particularly in childhood. Daniels et al. (18) evaluated this program by comparing latrine ownership in 803 cases of diarrhea in children presenting to health centers to 810 controls visiting the same clinics for reasons other than diarrhea. The mother's history of latrine ownership was validated in a substudy of about 200 study subjects by visiting the household. There was good agreement between the two types of measurement of latrine ownership. Latrine ownership had a protective effect of about 25% for diarrheal disease in these children.

9.2.2.8 Evaluation of health services. One of the points of emphasis of primary health care is that good primary care will prevent expensive hospitalization. In a case-control study from Bahrain, Malik et al. (19) compared cases that were hospitalized and controls of the same age and from the same neighborhood as to the use of a new health center in the township. The hypothesis was that use of the health center would be protective against hospital admission. The cases were higher utilizers of the health center than the controls, highlighting that the intervention tested (use of services of the health center) was not geared to prevent hospitalization. The health center was also a venue to channel patients to the hospital. Similar findings were reported in 1996 by Weinberger et al. (20) in a multicenter randomized, controlled trial at nine Veterans' Affairs Medical Centers where the intervention involved increased access to primary care through the use of close follow-up by a nurse and a primary care physician.

9.2.3 Strategies for Using Case-Control Studies to Evaluate Interventions

The case-control method should be considered for evaluation when we are studying adverse drug effects, rare outcomes, and when we can identify a population where the intervention is actively used or was used in the past.

The following are some design maneuvers that should be considered in developing a case-control study to evaluate interventions:

1. Define the outcome(s) to be prevented by this intervention clearly. Such a clear delineation will make our case definition much simpler.
2. Use tested definitions of outcomes and data collection procedures, if possible.
3. Select controls that are part of the population from where the cases are being drawn. This will allow us to have a comparison group that has a similar "opportunity for exposure" to the intervention as the cases.
4. Aim at introducing some random approach in the selection of the controls and cases (if sufficient numbers of cases are available).
5. Consider more than one group of controls for more than one manner of testing the hypothesis.
6. Compare the cases and the controls as to baseline characteristics and potential confounders.

7. Use identical data collection procedures for cases and controls.
8. Use a masked data collection procedure about exposures for both cases and controls.
9. Interview cases and controls simultaneously using a random approach to protect from biased inferences originating from secular trends.
10. Generate "active" data from alternative sources of information such as interviews, in addition to using "passive" data about exposure to the interventions.
11. Obtain as detailed information about exposure to medications and interventions as possible, including date of exposure, dose, and batch. When a medication is used chronically over several decades and the effect we are studying is of shorter duration, it is recommended that we define the exposed as *new* users of the drug consistent to our hypothesized mechanism of action, rather than as "prevalent" users (21).
12. Compare factors between the group exposed to the intervention and those who were not. This should be one of the first steps in the analysis of data, in addition to a case and control group comparison of the various characteristics and potential confounders, If the two groups of exposure are quite similar as to baseline characteristics and confounders, then our certainty about the findings is strengthened.
13. Try maneuvers for an independent replication and verification of the findings.

9.3 EVALUATING VACCINES AND VACCINATION PROGRAMS

The evaluation of vaccines and vaccination programs using the case-control method has been in use since the early 1980s (24). Some of the earliest case-control studies in this area have evaluated the effectiveness of BCG vaccination in populations with mixed vaccination status (25). In this application of the case-control design, the methods are relatively well standardized. The following are some specific areas of emphasis that one needs to consider in designing a case-control evaluation of vaccines and vaccination programs.

Definition of cases delineates the study population where the vaccine has been used. Our definition of cases of the disease that the vaccine will prevent has to be as specific and sensitive as possible. At times we may have to use laboratory confirmation for at least a subgroup of cases. It will be important to use some standardized definitions of cases used in prior studies to improve comparability of results with these prior studies.

Ascertainment of cases can be done through existing surveillance systems or using a more active search for new cases of the disease to be prevented.

Definition of controls. In addition to the previously cited basic guidelines for control selection, questions that need to be considered include whether people who are previously infected should be candidates for control selection. The answer to this question depends on the length of immunity imparted by the disease and the vaccine.

Ascertaining vaccination or exposure. Compared to a number of other case-control studies, these studies of the evaluation of a vaccine are able to evaluate vaccination status through records or other directly measured evidence. Recorded information does not just help validate vaccination status but can also potentially provide information on vaccine batch, dose, and date. For example, to assess BCG vaccination status one may interview cases and controls, one may check the BCG scar, and/or one may inspect the record of the study subject. In the upcoming example from Tanzania, different sources of information on exposure to the vaccine will provide different estimates of efficacy (26). Data collection about vaccination status needs to be independent from case-control selection or ascertainment. As stated previously, we need to compare the vaccinated and the nonvaccinated as to potential confounders to ascertain the validity of our inferences from the study.

Preventing bias. It is important that vaccination status does not influence detection of the disease that we are trying to prevent. Our case-control assessment should establish whether the vaccination status of a person did influence the case status. A frequently encountered issue is the choice of the population where such an assessment is being conducted. Do both vaccinated and nonvaccinated persons in the population have an equal chance of exposure to the infection (23)?

Stratification. As the effect of the vaccine may vary with the various forms of the disease, the analysis of the case-control study may include a stratified analysis by severity of cases to assess whether such differences affect our estimates of vaccine effectiveness. One needs to note that, in addition to the above, the effect of the vaccine may not be one of complete protection and that some vaccines may only make the disease manifestations milder. Thus, our case definition may have to be modified appropriately to include the severe forms only and we may need to consider forming another study subgroup to include people with the milder forms of the disease.

9.3.1 Efficacy Formulas

Although in a case-control study we are not able to calculate the RR, the OR may provide a valid approximation to it. Thus, it is possible to replace in the Greenwood-Yule formula RR with an OR. In certain epidemics a majority of the population may be affected with the disease, therefore, the rare disease assumption may not apply and the OR may not give us a close approximation of the RR. It may be worthwhile in such situations to consider a case-cohort approach for our evaluation. In a case-cohort approach we do not need to have the rare disease assumption since we are estimating the RR. Thus, Greenwood and Yule's formula would be applicable in a case-cohort analysis. More recently Orenstein et al. (23) proposed a formula that ascertains vaccine effectiveness (VE) using the two parameters of proportion of cases that have been vaccinated and the proportion of the population who are vaccinated.

Greenwood-Yule: VE = 1 − RR, in which RR is relative risk of disease association with vaccination (22).

Orenstein et al.: VE = $(p - c)/p(1 - c)$
where p is proportion of vaccinated in total population, and c is proportion of vaccinated in cases (23).

9.4 EXAMPLES OF INVESTIGATIONS

9.4.1 Measles in Tanzania

A concern of maintaining the potency of vaccines under difficult field circumstances led Killewo et al. (26) to assess the effectiveness of the measles vaccine in Dar Es Salam, Tanzania. A number of cases of measles in children were being reported to the health services, with a few giving a history of measles vaccination. A case-control study was set up to assess the efficacy of the vaccine that was in use. Cases with measles admitted to the university hospital were compared to four matched neighborhood controls per case as to measles vaccination status. Data were collected by interviewing the mothers as well as ascertaining vaccination status through the health card of the child. The efficacy of the vaccine reached expected levels (95%) when the strictest criteria for case definition and vaccination status were used. This led the investigators to conclude that the epidemic of measles observed in the community was not due to the lack of the potency of the vaccine.

9.4.2 Meningococcal Disease in Brazil

To control epidemic serogroup B meningococcal disease in the Sao Paulo region of Brazil during 1989 and 1990, an outer-membrane-protein-based serogroup B meningococcal vaccine was given to about 2.4 million children aged from three months to six years. De Moraes et al. (27) conducted a case-control study to estimate the efficacy of the vaccine in this same population. From a hospital-based surveillance system, 112 cases of meningococcal disease were identified and were matched on age and neighborhood to 409 controls. Estimated vaccine efficacy varied by age. The vaccine's efficacy was limited to children older than 48 months and to adults.

9.4.3 Japanese Encephalitis in Nepal

In July, 1999, a single dose of live attenuated Japanese encephalitis vaccine was given to available children in the Terai region of Nepal. In 2000, this same population had another seasonal exposure to the same encephalitis virus. For Ohrr et al. (28) this was an opportunity to test the long-term protective effect of the vaccine. Their cases were 35 serologically confirmed cases of hospitalized Japanese encephalitis and of these only one was vaccinated in 1999, while in 430 age-sex-matched village controls, 234 (54.4%) were vaccinated. The unbiased estimate of the OR was 0.0155 (95% CI: 0.0004–0.0986). The protective effect of the vaccine after 12 to 15 months was 98.5% (95% CI: 90.1–99.2)

9.5 CONCLUSION

The case-control method can be used in a sequential design or as part of a continuous surveillance program that monitors the effectiveness of a vaccine periodically in a population (see Chapter 11). It is also a useful method to continuously ascertain potential side effects of a vaccine or therapeutic interventions in a controlled environment. In such a design and as part of the routine surveillance program, a control is selected without the outcome(s) from the base population whenever a case with the disease or with the side effect is identified. On a periodic basis one compares these cases and controls to assess whether there are changes in the effectiveness of the intervention or significant side effects that one needs to address or take preventive action.

The case-control design is a very effective tool for evaluating a number of interventions and programs. It is important, however, to minimize different types of biases that may affect our inferences. The method should not be used as a substitute for controlled experimental trials when we have the need for such trials and the resources to conduct them properly. We need also to consider that, as part of a quality assurance and surveillance program, we may design an ongoing case-control evaluation that assesses performance of health services on an ongoing basis.

REFERENCES

1. Habicht JP, Victora CG, Vaughan JP. Evaluation designs for adequacy, plausibility and probability of public health programme performance and impact. *Int J Epidemiol.* 199;28:10-18.
2. Christie CDC, Marx ML, Marchant CD, Reising SF. The 1993 epidemic of pertussis in Cincinnati. Resurgence of disease in a highly immunized population of children. *N Engl J Med.* 1994;331:16-21.
3. Herman J. Experiment and observation. *Lancet.* 1994;344:1209-1210.
4. Jick H, Rodriguez LAG, Perez-Gutthann S. Principles of epidemiological research on adverse and beneficial drug effects. *Lancet.* 1998;352:1767-1770.
5. Steinwachs DM, Wu AW, Cagney KA. Outcomes research and quality of care. In: Spiker B, ed. *Quality of Life and Pharmacoeconomics in Clinical Trials,* 2nd ed. Philadelphia: Lippincott-Raven Publishers; 1996:747-752.
6. Selby JW. Case-control evaluations of treatment and program efficacy. *Epidemiol Rev.* 1994;16:90-101.
7. Marks HM. Rigorous uncertainty: why RA Fisher is important. *Int J Epidemiol.* 2003;32:932-937.
8. Smith PG. Evaluating interventions against tropical diseases. *Int J Epidemiol.* 1987;16:159-166.
9. Victora CG, Habicht JP, Bryce J. Evidence based public health: moving beyond randomized trials. *Am J Public Health.* 2004;94:400-405.
10. Sivak-Sears NR, Schwartzbaum JA, Miike R, Moghadassi M, Wrensch M. Case-control study of nonsteroidal anti-inflammatory drugs and glioblastoma multiforme. *Am J Epidemiol.* 2004;159:1131-1139.
11. Hellman S, Hellman DS. Of mice but not men. Problems of the randomized clinical trial. *N Engl J Med.* 1991; 324:1585-1589.
12. Jick H, Vessey MP. Case-control studies in the evaluation of drug-induced illness. *Am J Epidemiol.* 1978;107:1-7.
13. Tonascia J, Gordis L, Schmerler H. Retrospective evidence favoring use of anticoagulants for myocardial infarctions. *N Engl J Med.* 1975;292:1362-1366.
14. Modan B, Shani M, Schor S, Modan M. Reduction of hospital mortality from acute myocardial infarction by anticoagulant therapy. *N Engl J Med.* 1975;292:1359-1362.
15. Levy M. Aspirin use in patients with major upper gastrointestinal bleeding and peptic-ulcer disease. A report from the Boston Collaborative Drug Surveillance Program, Boston University Medical Center. *N Engl J Med.* May 23, 1974;290(21):1158-1162.
16. Kirsh VA, Kreiger N, Cotterchio M, Sloan M, Theis B. Nonsteroidal anti-inflammatory drug use and breast cancer risk: subgroup findings. *Am J Epidemiol.* 2007;166:709-716.

17. Cook MN, Olshan AF, Guess HA, et al. Maternal medication use and neuroblastoma in offspring. *Am J Epidemiol.* 2004;159:721-731.

18. Daniels DL, Cousens SN, Makoae LN, Feachem RG. A case-control study of the impact of improved sanitation on diarrhea morbidity in Lesotho.: *Bull WHO* 1990;68:455-463.

19. Malik Clarisse. Hospitalization related to Isa Town health center visits in Bahrain. Thesis, Department of Epidemiology and Biostatistics, American University of Beirut, 1977.

20. Weinberger M, Oddone EZ, Henderson WG. Does increased access to primary care reduce hospital readmissions? *N Engl J Med.* 1996;334:1441-1447.

21. Ray WA. Evaluating medication effects outside of clinical trials: new-drug user designs. *Am J Epidemiol.* 2003;158:915-920.

22. Greenwood M, Yule GU. The statistics of anti-typhoid and anti-cholera inoculations and the interpretation of such statistics in general. *Proceedings of the Royal Society of Medicine* (Epidemiology) 1915;8:113-190.

23. Orenstein WA, Bernier RH, Dondero TJ, et al. Field evaluation of vaccine efficacy. *Bull WHO.* 1985;63:1055-1068.

24. Comstock GW. Evaluating vaccination effectiveness and vaccine efficacy by means of case-control studies. *Epidemiol Rev.* 1994;16:77-89.

25. Smith PG. Retrospective assessment of the effectiveness of BCG vaccination against tuberculosis using the case-control method. *Tubercle.* 1982;62:23-35.

26. Killewo J, Makwaya C, Munubhi E, Mpembeni R. The protective effect of measles vaccine in Dar Es Salam, Tanzania. *Int J Epidemiol.* 1991;20:508-514.

27. De Moraes JC, Perkins BA, Camargo MCC, et al. Protective efficacy of a serogroup B meningococcal vaccine in Sao Paulo, Brazil. *Lancet.* Oct 31, 1992;340:1074-1078.

28. Ohrr H, Tandan JB, Mo Sohn Y, Shin SH, Pradhan DP, Halstead SB. Effect of single dose of SA 14-14-2 vaccine 1 year after immunization in Nepalese children with Japanese encephalitis: a case-control study. *Lancet.* 2005;366:1375-1378.

10

APPLICATIONS: EVALUATION
OF SCREENING PROGRAMS

Haroutune K. Armenian

OUTLINE

This chapter aims to

1. review various approaches to the evaluation of screening programs;
2. describe the advantages of the case-control method for the evaluation of screening programs; and
3. discuss specific problems in the use of the case-control method in evaluating screening programs.

10.1 BASIC PRINCIPLES OF EARLY DISEASE DETECTION

The following brief review of some principles of early disease detection should facilitate our discussion of the evaluation of screening programs. When initiating a screening program, the following should be considered:

1. The condition sought should be *highly prevalent* in the screened population.
2. The disease to be screened should have *serious consequences.*
3. An *acceptable treatment* for patients with the disease should exist. This treatment should be more effective when applied to the screen-detected stage of the disease than when applied after symptoms have led to diagnosis.
4. There should be *a detectable preclinical phase* (DPCP).
5. There should be a *suitable test* with
   a. adequate sensitivity and specificity,
   b. low cost,
   c. convenience and ease of administering, and
   d. absence of morbidity from the test.

As we assess the effectiveness of screening programs it is important to be familiar with the concepts of *lead-time, length of DPCP* of the disease, and *referral bias.*

10.1.1 Discussion and Examples

The *detectable preclinical phase* (DPCP) is the period of time where one is able to detect the disease prior to the development of clinical symptoms and signs or prior to clinical onset of the disease. As a concept, DPCP is theoretical and difficult to measure for most diseases, but it helps us to appreciate the intricacies of evaluating a screening program. The longer the DPCP, the higher the probability that a screening test will be able to detect the disease successfully.

DPCP depends on the disease under consideration, its natural history, and the *sensitivity* of the instruments used for detection. DPCP is also delimited by the *critical points* in the natural history of the disease. As a concept critical points are points of no return. Past these points one is not able (with the interventions available at the time) to move the patient back to an earlier stage of the disease in its natural history. Thus, beyond the critical point for DPCP, one will not be able to influence the natural history of the disease through early detection or screening. There may, however, be another critical point for curable disease, but past the critical point of the detectable curable preclinical phase one may not be able to have any impact on the natural history of the condition through therapeutic means. The duration of the DPCP can be crudely estimated by dividing prevalence with incidence of such cases.

Although such a test may be able to detect the disease early with a high level of sensitivity and specificity, we need to evaluate any screening program because it may not improve the natural history of the disease if the interventions following the detection are not effective. Thus the evaluation of a screening program goes beyond the validation of the test as to its sensitivity, specificity, and other test characteristics. These test parameters assess the disease detection process rather than the impact of the test on the disease load in the community. *It is important to demonstrate that screening prevents morbidity, disability, and mortality.*

Like any other intervention, there are two levels of evaluation:

1. *Efficacy.* Does the screening procedure work?
2. *Effectiveness.* What is the usefulness of the screening program as it is applied in the community and in real life?

The evaluation of a screening program combines an assessment of the joint effect of: (1) the *use* of the screening test for the detection of subclinical disease, and (2) the *management* of the patient following detection and the impact of treatment on the natural history of the disease.

Thus, *the efficacy and effectiveness of a screening program cannot be larger than the sensitivity of the screening test used.* This is because cases of the disease that were missed by the screening test will not benefit from the program.

A screening test may also have some side effects, and these may not be innocuous. As with any intervention, one needs to evaluate adverse effects of the screening program beyond its positive impact.

Finally, considering that a screening program uses sizable resources, a *cost benefit evaluation* of the program is mandatory prior to generalizing the procedure. For example, the rapid diffusion of serum prostate-specific antigen (PSA) testing in clinical practice in the late 1980s and early 1990s as a screening test for prostate cancer resulted in a dramatic epidemic of prostate cancer. The massive use of the PSA test occurred without the appropriate population-based evaluation as a screening test with regard for its value for reducing prostate cancer mortality (1). In a 10-year retrospective cohort study among 2,400 women, Elmore et al. (2) assessed the impact of false positive mammograms for breast cancer. One-third of the women screened had abnormal test results needing additional evaluation over the 10-year period even though no breast cancer was present. The authors estimated that for every $100 spent for screening, an additional $33 was spent to evaluate the false positive results.

A strong interest developed in the 1960s and 1970s in initiating multiphasic screening as preventive public health programs. Such programs involved testing individuals for a number of parameters with the understanding that such a workup of the individual will help to identify illnesses early and help take preventive action. A classic example of such a program that has been evaluated through a randomized controlled trial was the South-East London Screening Study conducted by Walter Holland and colleagues (3). In this study, 7,729 individuals aged between 40 and 64 were randomly allocated into either a screening or a control group and followed until 1972–1973. The intervention group received multiphasic screening that included questionnaires, anthropometry, vision and hearing testing, chest X-ray, lung function tests, electrocardiogram, blood pressure, blood tests, stools testing for occult blood, and a standard examination by a physician. The control group was followed through their usual sources of care. Both groups were invited to undergo a health survey in 1972–1973. No significant differences between the two study groups were evident in any of the outcome measures nine years after the initiation of the study. These results cast doubt about the effectiveness of the multiphasic screening programs initiated at the time. The authors estimated that in 1976 prices to implement such a program in the whole of the United Kingdom would have cost annually 142 million pounds.

10.2 APPROACHES FOR EVALUATING SCREENING PROGRAMS

10.2.1 Overview

The effectiveness of screening programs can be evaluated using a variety of epidemiological methods.

The gold standard for evaluation is again the randomized controlled trial. Individuals are randomly assigned to the screening procedure or no screening and the outcome of the program is assessed in both groups. As with all randomized trials, the design aims at minimizing selection bias and the effect of confounders. The outcome is usually mortality or disability, since it is expected that the screening will improve the natural history of the disease. Classic randomized controlled trials of screening evaluation include the Hospital Insurance Plan of New York trial in the 1960s on the effectiveness of mammography (4). Women enrolled in the Health Insurance Program were assigned at random to screening by mammography and control groups and were followed for a decade. The death rate from breast cancer was higher in the control group when compared to the screened group.

A number of difficulties can arise in setting up randomized experimental trials to evaluate screening programs. These trials are usually very *expensive* and sometimes take a *number of decades* to ascertain appropriately the outcomes of interest. For a rare outcome, these trials may require a *large sample* for the study population, and the original screening procedure may be *technically outdated* by the time the results of the trial are published. It should also be noted that a number of screening procedures may be used extensively in the community as a *clinical-detection* procedure prior to the development of the trial.

10.2.2 Nonexperimental Approaches to the Evaluation of Screening Programs

These include

1. Studies of *time trends* in populations where screening has been established for a number of years. The evidence for the effectiveness of Pap smear screening for cervical cancer was initially based on such data. Time trends of mortality from cervical cancer had started decreasing dramatically in the U.S. in a number of states following the introduction of Pap smears for cervical cancer screening. This is the model of a before-and-after comparison and does not necessarily consider the potential role of confounders in such comparisons.

2. Studies of *geographic comparisons* of areas with different intensities of screening. This approach also has the same shortcoming of not considering a number of confounders that may explain the differences in outcome.

3. *Comparison of individuals.* The two main analytic designs of epidemiology can be used to assess the effectiveness of screening programs. In a *cohort* design we identify individuals who have undergone or are undergoing screening: the mortality, disability, and complications from the disease of interest in this group are compared to the same outcomes from the same condition in a group of individuals who are not screened. In a *case-control* design, cases of death or other adverse outcomes are compared to controls that are alive, as to the frequency of past "exposure" to screening in both groups. For both of these observational designs one needs to address the issue of selection bias. People who are

screened may differ in a number of ways from persons who are not screened. Compared to the randomized clinical trial, a cohort study aimed at assessing a screening program can evaluate evolving protocols of screening as these are applied in the population over time. Also, in situations where a screening test such as the PSA is introduced into clinical practice without the appropriate experimental evidence, a cohort or case-control study may be the best alternative for evaluation.

10.3 THE CASE-CONTROL METHOD FOR EVALUATING SCREENING PROGRAMS

10.3.1 Overview

A number of studies have been published using the case-control method to evaluate screening programs. Some of these tackle methodological issues which are particular to the evaluation of screening programs and will be discussed here in more detail.

The starting point of such an evaluative study is finding an appropriate population where the study will be conducted. There should be "*opportunity for exposure*" to the screening procedure in the selected community. Those who are targeted by the screening program should not have differential access because of risk factors to develop the outcome that the screening procedure is aiming to prevent. For example, if smokers are particularly selected for Pap smear screening for cervical cancer, then we may end up with a biased estimate of the effect of the screening test because smoking is a risk factor for cervical cancer. It is also essential to select a population and a time period for that population when there is *variability* in the use of the screening procedure. It is not possible to be able to make any inferences about the effectiveness of Pap smear screening in a community where every woman gets the procedure to the same extent.

Advantages of the case-control method include its ability to assess the *frequency* of screening and to measure the effect of *variations over time and place* and of *technical changes* of screening procedures on the outcome. Sometimes a case-control study can also evaluate a number of procedural differences within one study.

As our evaluation of a screening program involves not just the early detection of the disease but also the treatment that will follow to improve the natural history of the condition, a subgroup analysis in a case-control study can observe the effect of treatment differentials that follow the detection of the disease. In such an analysis we may be able to stratify the cases and controls by screening status and assess the effect of treatment in those subgroups. When a majority of the target population is screened through clinical services—for example, with the prostate-specific antigen in some communities—our study may focus on the question of whether we are able to influence the natural history of prostate cancer in PSA screen-detected prostate cancer.

Considering the importance of confounders for our inferences, we need to ascertain that the cases and controls are selected from the same base population. Thus, we hope to establish some level of comparability of cases and controls with regard to the various confounders. However, it is critical for studies evaluating interventions—as discussed previously—to establish some level of comparability of the exposed and nonexposed groups, with the purpose of testing for opportunity for exposure, as well as level of control of confounders. Case-control studies that have a high level of comparability of the exposure comparison groups as to known confounders may be closer to efficacy studies, in addition to studying effectiveness.

10.3.2 Definition of Outcome or Case Definition

The definition of the outcome in a case-control study of program evaluation is dependent on the formulation of the *objectives of the program*. Is this program aimed at preventing incidence of the disease, mortality, or disability as a result of its complications? For example, screening for hypertension as a procedure aims at preventing the secondary complications of hypertension. A case-control study of the impact of screening for hypertension will have as its outcome incident stroke or kidney failure. Thus, in such a *primary prevention* study, our cases will be incident stroke or incident kidney failure patients. In a *secondary prevention* screening program for detection of early stages of cancer, we aim at preventing death or the advanced and disabling forms of the disease; the cases will be people who die from the cancer or develop the metastatic forms of the disease.

In a case-control study, it is important to focus on incident outcomes to prevent incidence-prevalence bias. Thus, uncomplicated cases of the disease identified as a result of screening should not be considered as cases unless they develop the outcome(s) we are trying to prevent by the screening program (disability, complications, and death).

People with the disease, detected by screening are potential beneficiaries of secondary prevention of death and complications. These are persons identified during the *detectable preclinical period* of the disease. By including such persons as cases, one may underestimate the effectiveness of the screening program. If screening is beneficial, then its impact should occur during this detectable preclinical period by detecting such disease early.

Although, prevention of mortality and improved survival is the eventual yardstick against which a screening program needs to be tested, a number of situations may arise, as in cervical cancer; with low mortality rates and the sample size for a case-control evaluation of such screening may be very limited. In addition, one may be interested in assessing the role of the screening program in preventing the primary disease or incident cases by detecting antecedents to clinical illness. Weiss (5) has proposed that in diseases where it is possible to identify such antecedent stages to the disease through screening, one may consider doing a case-control assessment of the test to measure its impact as a primary prevention of the disease. In such a study one needs to know the length of the predisease phase and the timing of the screening tests that are applied in our study groups.

10.3.3 *Control Selection*

To select appropriate controls, we need to understand the measure that the control group will provide: the frequency of screening procedures in a group of people without the outcome (i.e., without disability, death, or complications) from the same base population as the cases. Thus, although the need to provide a high measure of comparability to the cases is important for minimizing confounding, the control group also has a role in providing us with an assessment of what happens with regard to screening in the population. The screening history of the controls should reflect the history of screening of the base population.

The selection of controls is best done by sampling directly from the population from which the cases are selected. Thus, as in other case-control studies, controls can be selected from available population registries or membership lists of people enrolled in the same health-care system (6).

As in other types of case-control studies, we need to assure that the screened and nonscreened persons in the study come from the same base population (see Section on Definition of outcome).

Our definition of controls needs to include all members of the base population without the adverse outcome or death as candidates to be selected as controls. Hence, if our case definition is death with the disease, our control group may theoretically include persons with the disease who are alive.

10.3.4 *Exposure Assessment*

A number of sources of exposure information about screening can be useful, including personal interviews, and medical and screening records.

Information collected from records may be more complete and accurate than individual histories obtained through interview. Sometimes the medical record may be the only source of valid data since the study subject may have died a few months following the development of the disease.

Information needs to be as complete as possible and according to a standardized data gathering processes. Every study needs to validate its screening exposure information systematically.

10.3.5 Collecting Data

The following are some guidelines for collecting data on screening from cases and controls:

1. The *time period selected* for obtaining screening procedure exposure information should be similar for cases and controls. This period needs to encompass and focus on the DPCP when the procedure is potentially beneficial.
2. Evaluation of screening needs to *assess the period of time* during which screening was conducted. The issue of *timing* may be very important to prenatal screening, since it may be possible to detect the disease during a limited window in the pregnancy. Such issues of timing are also very important for detecting the disease at the detectable preclinical phase. It may be best to test various preclinical periods to identify the time when observed differences are maximized, which is to be expected because the screening test will have its maximum impact during DPCP.
3. It is necessary to *validate that every reported procedure* was used for screening purposes and not for diagnostic purposes. Misclassification of the same test used for diagnostic purposes decreases assessment of the effectiveness of the screening procedure. An examination of medical records may allow one to ascertain the purpose of the test. In a number of situations, this can be difficult to assess. Weiss (7) reviewed this issue and the biases it may potentially lead to and recommended that (1) among persons with symptoms that clearly are the result of the disease and that lead to a test, the test should not be considered as screening; (2) if the test was conducted following some symptoms but these symptoms are not related to the disease to be screened, dual analyses can be done that include and exclude such persons and their tests; and (3) if the test results for a symptomatic person are negative for the disease, subsequent tests in that person can be considered as screens.
4. *A screening test is to be followed by diagnostic validation* in almost all cases. Thus, the use of the diagnostic evaluation

following a positive screening test allows validation of the screening and of the initiation of a therapeutic process. One should also expect that a number of therapeutic or other interventions will be started at that time.

10.3.6 Confounding

As with any study, an important concern for controlling for confounders in a program evaluation of screening is their *correct definition*. Assessment of confounding needs to focus on the potential alternative explanations of the observed relationship that other factors can provide. The relationship under scrutiny is between the screening procedure and the adverse outcome of the disease that the screening is designed to prevent. Thus, some of the risk factors for the disease may not be relevant at all as confounders for such an evaluation. Sexual activity may be a risk factor for cervical cancer but it may not be relevant in a study of the evaluation of Pap smear screening. Access to health care may be more of a concern as a confounder in such a study.

10.4 EXAMPLES

The following are two examples of case-control evaluations of screening programs. The first is based on data from an HMO and the second is a case-control evaluation of a population-based screening program.

10.4.1 A Case-Control Study of Screening Sigmoidoscopy and Mortality from Colorectal Cancer (8)

Objective. To assess the efficacy of screening by the use of the rigid sigmoidoscope in reducing mortality from colon cancer at sites within reach of the screening instrument (last portion of the colorectum).

Outcome measurement. Deaths from colon cancer at sites within reach of the sigmoidoscope. These deaths are identified through the medical records and death certificates.

Case definition. Persons with the outcome that the screening program is intended to prevent. In this particular situation, cases are people who died from colorectal cancer of the descending colon-rectum.

Controls. These are persons who do not have the outcome described above. In this study the authors used two types of controls: those from the same HMO population without the outcome and who were alive at the time of the death of the matched case (incidence density sampling), and a set of controls from patients who died from colorectal cancers that were in locations outside the reach of the sigmoidoscope.

Exposure measurement. Standardized data collection methods and a comparable period of assessment of screening for cases and controls were used. The screening tests that were considered were those conducted prior to the diagnosis of colon cancer. Two blinded independent reviewers of the medical records classified the tests as to whether the test was for screening or for diagnostic purposes.

Assessment of confounding. Several confounding factors were assessed including history of adenomatous polyp, a prior family history of colorectal cancer, and a diagnosis of ulcerative colitis and hereditary polyposis before the diagnosis of the fatal cancer. These factors could lead to both increased screening and also increased risk of the outcome of death from colorectal cancer.

Results. Only 8.8 % of the 261 cases of death from colorectal cancer had undergone sigmoidoscopy compared to 24.2% of the 868 controls (matched odds ratio (OR) 0.30; 95% CI: 0.19–0.48). The OR following multivariate adjustment for potential confounding was 0.41 (95% CI: 0.25–0.69). This finding of protection was maintained even if the most recent sigmoidoscopic examination was 9 to 10 years before the diagnosis of colorectal cancer. By contrast, for the 268 subjects with fatal colon cancer above the reach of the sigmoidoscope compared to their controls, the adjusted OR was 0.96 (95% CI: 0.61–1.50). "The specificity of the negative association for cancer within the reach of the sigmoidoscope is consistent with a true efficacy of screening rather than a confounding by unmeasured selection factors" (2).

Conclusions. The authors concluded that screening by the use of sigmoidoscopy can reduce mortality from colorectal cancer in the rectum and distal colon and that screening every 10 years may be as efficacious as more frequent screening.

10.4.2 A Case-Control Study of the Efficacy of a Nonrandomized Breast Cancer-Screening Program in Florence (Italy) (9)

Objective. To evaluate the efficacy of a population-based screening program for breast cancer that was started in a rural area near Florence, Italy, in 1970 and that offered mammographic screening every 2.5 years to all women aged 40 to 70 years of age. A case-control study was conducted.

Outcome measurement and case definition. All female residents in the screening area certified as having died from breast cancer in the years 1977–1984 were considered as cases. From a total of 143 women identified from death certificates, only 57 were eligible as cases: 45 were not eligible to participate in the screening program because of age. For another 38 women, a diagnosis of breast cancer was established prior to an invitation to participate in the screening program, and in 3 others the date of diagnosis of the breast cancer could not be established.

Controls. Each case was matched on year of birth and residence to five randomly selected controls that were eligible for the screening program.

Exposure measurement. Through the use of computerized screening records, data were collected on all 57 cases and 285 matched controls. Similar periods of time were considered for both the case and the five controls for assessing frequency of mammographic screening. For example, if the case moved to the area after the program had begun, only tests that were done after the case arrived and before the diagnosis was established were considered for both the case and the controls.

Assessment of confounding. Control of confounding was partially achieved by very close matching of the cases and controls on year of birth and residence.

Results. The overall OR for mammographic screening was 0.53 (95% CI: 0.29–0.95). The adjusted OR was 0.57 (95% CI: 0.35–0.92) for women screened only once and 0.32 (95% CI: 0.20–0.52) for women screened at least twice during the study period. When the analysis was stratified by age, no significant protective effect was shown for women below the age of 50 years.

Conclusions. The authors demonstrated a significant trend for increased protective effect with increasing number of mammographic examinations for screening for breast cancer in this population-based program.

10.5 CONCLUSIONS

The case-control method offers a number of advantages for the evaluation of screening programs compared to other methods of evaluation:

1. Compared to randomized controlled trials, it provides an assessment of the effectiveness of the screening procedure in normal operating conditions. It provides an evaluation of *effectiveness* of the program rather than its efficacy.
2. As a procedure it is *efficient* and cost-effective.
3. The method provides an opportunity to assess the impact of a number of *other factors* in addition to the screening procedure. It allows us to identify subgroups in the population who may do better with the procedure. One can study confounders and a number of interactions.

4. Considering the variability with which some screening procedures may be applied in the population, one may be able to analyze the effect of the *frequency* of screening and the differences in
   time intervals between two procedures.
5. The case-control method may be able to assess the effect of the
   changes in the screening procedures over time with evolving
   technology.

It is possible that an evaluation of a screening program may be *part
of an etiological case-control study.* Hoffman et al. (10) conducted an
assessment of Pap smear screening in a case-control study of the association of hormonal contraceptives and invasive cervical cancer in South
Africa. Incident cases (n = 524) of invasive cervical cancer were matched
on age, race, and residence to 1,540 controls from the same tertiary
care hospital. The investigators carefully selected control diagnoses that
minimized selection biases. The OR of invasive cervical cancer among
women who ever had a Pap smear was 0.3 (95% CI: 0.3–0.4). The OR
further declined with increasing number of smears. The Pap smear was
protective even after an interval of over 15 years.

REFERENCES

1. Potosky AL, Miller BA, Albertsen PC, Kramer BS. The role of increasing
   detection in the rising incidence of prostate cancer. *JAMA.* 1995;273:
   548-552.
2. Elmore JG, Barton MB, Moceri VM, Polk S, Arena PJ, Fletcher SW. Ten year
   risk of false positive screening mammograms and clinical breast examination.
   N Engl J Med. 1998;338:1089-1096.
3. The South-East London Screening Study Group. A controlled trial of multiphasic screening in middle age: results of the South-East London Screening
   Study. *Int J Epidemiol.* 1977;6:357-363.
4. Shapiro S, Venet W, Strax P, Venet L. *Periodic Screening for Breast Cancer:
   the Health Insurance Plan Project and Its Sequelae, 1963–1986.* Baltimore,
   MD: Johns Hopkins University Press; 1988.
5. Weiss NS. Case-control studies of the efficacy of screening tests designed to
   prevent the incidence of cancer. *Am J Epidemiol.* 1999;149:1-4.
6. Weiss NS. Application of the case-control method in the evaluation of screening. *Epidemiol Rev.* 1994;16:103-108.
7. Weiss NS. Analysis of case-control studies of the efficacy of screening for
   cancer: how should we deal with tests done in persons with symptoms? *Am
   J Epidemiol.* 1998;147:1099-1102.
8. Selby JV, Friedman GD, Quesenberry CP, Weiss NS. A case-control study of
   screening sigmoidoscopy and mortality from colorectal cancer. *N Engl J Med.*
   1992;326:653-657.

9. Palli D, Roselli Del Turco M, Bulatti E, et al. A case-control study of the efficacy of a nonrandomized breast cancer-screening program in Florence (Italy). *Int J Cancer.* 1986;38:501-504.
10. Hoffman M, Cooper D, Carrara H, et al. Limited Pap screening associated with reduced risk of cervical cancer in South Africa. *Int J Epidemiol.* 2003;32:573-577.

11

OTHER APPLICATIONS

*Haroutune K. Armenian
and Miriam Khlat*

OUTLINE

This chapter will describe a number of applications of the case-control method in various problem-solving situations. There is a broad spectrum of such applications of the case-control method. This presentation complements the earlier chapters on applications of the method. In dealing with these applications one needs to also consider other case-based designs as described in Chapter 5. Some of these designs may provide a better fit to these applications than the classic case-control approach.

11.1 SURVEILLANCE AND HEALTH INFORMATION SYSTEMS USING THE CASE-CONTROL METHOD

In the earlier chapter on the use of the case-control method in evaluation we noted that the method can be used for evaluating the quality of medical care by comparing patients with adverse outcomes of care (cases) to patients with positive outcomes (controls) as to the care and interventions they received. An analysis of the comparison will help modify patient care and improve outcomes. Below we describe this use of the case-control method as well as discuss using the case-control approach to develop a system of data processing that could be a useful tool for decision making at the clinical level.

The case-control method combined with a process of surveillance of outcomes can be an effective investigative tool that can provide critical information for decision making in, for example, communicable disease control, monitoring of adverse drug or vaccine outcomes, and quality assurance programs.

The method is of sequential design and can be part of a continuous surveillance program that monitors various outcomes. In such a design and as part of the routine surveillance program, a control(s) is selected without the outcome(s) from the base population when a case with the disease or side effect is identified. On a periodic basis one compares these cases and controls to assess whether changes have occurred in the effectiveness of the intervention or if there are significant side effects that need to be addressed or require taking preventive action. We need also to consider that as part of a quality assurance and surveillance program we may design an ongoing case-control evaluation that assesses performance of health services on a continuous basis.

For example, as part of such a surveillance and investigation system, one may identify serious side effects of a new vaccine and investigate each case of a person with side effects, comparing characteristics to persons who received the vaccine but who did not develop any serious side effects. Through this comparison, we hope to identify those characteristics that may be associated with or lead to these side effects, either through an interaction mechanism or through the circumstances of the intervention with the vaccine.

11.1.1 *Approaches to Decision Making*

In this section we illustrate one such application of this approach using quality assurance in medical care as a potential model. Prior to describing the system a theoretical framework for decision making will be discussed.

Health-care organizations need to assess outcomes of care as an ongoing activity. When a problem is identified, such as a possible serious side effect or a complication, two approaches may be considered for selecting a course of action:

1. Identify all the potential causes of the problem and embark on as many interventions as resources would allow. In this situation, "corrective" interventions are instituted based on antecedent knowledge and experience with similar circumstances, and with no specific diagnosis established. For example a major allergic reaction in a patient may lead the managing physicians to take a number of actions such as changing or stopping all new medications, and investigating a number of potential causes of this allergic reaction such as food eaten or equipment used. This approach does not identify a specific cause but addresses all possible causes of the allergic reaction.

2. Conduct a review of the records of a group of cases with the problem and get the professionals try to gain insights as to the causes of the adverse outcome. A certain level of judgment can be applied in this approach by comparing subgroups of various outcomes. This is the approach of the case-series when one is trying to make sense and find the cause(s) of the serious side effect from the cumulated information on similar cases that have occurred thus far.

11.1.2 *Levels of Data*

Information systems established in many health-care organizations are akin to epidemiologic surveillance systems that monitor the occurrence of certain conditions and investigate the problems as they are identified in the community. Most hospitals and health-care agencies institute two types of reviews and use data at two different levels:

At the *policy and institutional management* level, decisions are made based in part on routine statistical information systems. Data on success rates or utilization patterns that are included in the periodic statistical report are commonly used at the strategic level of the organization. The major advantage of the statistical report or information is that it can relate to a denominator and can help us to compare rates of particular outcomes of interest across time or across place and systems. Thus, one can compare the case fatality rates or complications in patients at more than one hospital or at the same institution during different time periods, if data collection procedures are similar. However, there are many limitations of these information systems, including issues of *validity and reliability* of the data and lack of appropriate *level of detail* for proper analysis.

At the *operational level* of patient care, the decision process needs case information. Of interest are sentinel outcomes such as untimely deaths or unexplained length-of-stay extensions. Thus, case-based information is essential for monitoring and evaluation at the operational level. The monitoring of cases or sentinel events allows an in-depth investigation of all potential factors that contribute to the development of the event and could lead to a more timely assessment and intervention. Such case or case-series data are generated as part of active reviews of the records of patients with various outcomes or diagnoses of interest or as part of ongoing patient care.

Using the case-control method as an investigative tool, one can link an existing health information system to a case-control method of analysis by generating data about a group of controls as the cases are being identified and investigated. The information from the individual cases and their controls could provide direct feedback at the operational level, while the estimates of risk from the case-control analysis can be the basis for a number of policy and strategic decisions. Beyond the routine analysis of statistical data such a system will provide a diagnostic tool for the institution in its investigation of inappropriate processes of care. Thus, the case-control method as part of the surveillance system of outcomes allows us to identify well-defined outcomes and to investigate various determinants of these outcomes.

11.1.3 *Steps in the Development of the Model*

This proposed model will generate the needed information for evaluating various services, monitoring sentinel events, and allowing special investigations of outcomes of interest.

1. The first step is one of reviewing the available data and deciding on the list of outcomes to be monitored. For example, which complications of treatment are of interest? Are there any sentinel outcomes that need to be identified as they occur?

2. For each of the sentinel events decisions are made on diagnostic criteria and tests that will validate these outcomes.
3. A control is selected without the outcome of interest for each of the sentinel events. Cases and controls are investigated by using the same diagnostic tests. Case and control data are recorded and cumulated over time.
4. Cases and controls are reviewed on a regular basis and inferences are made as an ongoing activity.
5. Case-control analyses are conducted on a regular basis as the sample size allows.

11.1.4 The Advantages of the Model

The advantages are listed below:

- This model links directly outcomes to process of care.
- Compared to the traditional methods of quality of care assessment that are based on a case-series, the case-control method has the major advantage of providing an analysis of both outliers (cases) and inliers (controls).
- The model provides useful information for evaluation at both strategic and operational levels.
- The medical professionals delivering the service are direct participants in the decisions as well as the operation of the system.
- Judgment of the effectiveness of the model is based on well-tested scientific methods that allow inferences which may have implications beyond the health-care facility under consideration.
- The method allows the use of multivariate analyses as a routine. Thus, one is able to assess the simultaneous effect of a number of determinants for the outcome under consideration.
- The medical professionals decide independently on the effectiveness of interventions from within their own system rather than only on information generated by others.
- By its sequential sampling of cases and controls the approach uses a more efficient sampling approach (1), as well as an incident density selection of controls.

11.1.5 Case Studies

The following are two examples of the potential applications of this model:

Hospital mortality study. Upon review of mortality statistics at the state level, it was reported that a particular inner city hospital had case fatality rates in the upper quartile of the distribution, compared with the other hospitals in the state. The medical chief of staff of the hospital was interested in finding the underlying reasons for the higher rate, and a case-control analysis of available Medicare data from this hospital was conducted. Considering that one of the most important in-hospital fatal outcomes was Myocardial Infarction (MI), cases were deaths with MI, and controls were patients with MI who were discharged alive. Cases and controls were compared as to sociodemographic characteristics, risk factors, disease severity indicators, treatments received, and procedures undergone. Following adjustment for various severity and sociodemographic confounders, a major difference that emerged between the cases and controls involved the procedures undergone in the hospital. However, a critical review of the coding of these procedures that were done for Medicare reporting purposes revealed that the coding was very much influenced by whether the patients survived. This compromised the ability of the investigators to pass on an unbiased judgment about the data and the case-control analysis since exposure definition was very much influenced by the case status for coding purposes.

Case investigation for cancer prevention. The County Health Officer of a sparsely populated area was interested in establishing a system for monitoring and investigating cancers similar to a system already in place for communicable diseases. Thus, elements of a test system were tried whereby every new reported case of cancer would be investigated using a questionnaire including questions regarding number of potential exposures as well as methods of detection and management. A neighborhood control without cancer would be matched on age and gender and would undergo a similar investigation using the interview questionnaire. Data would be analyzed periodically for any salient patterns of differences between the cases of cancer and their controls. Based on such analysis, the Health Department should be able to identify special subgroups that need preventive intervention, as well as to identify failures of the health-care system in dealing with such patients. Although a number of the instruments were developed and pretested, lack of funds did not allow the formal institutionalization of this model.

The above illustrate the potential wealth of applications of the case-control method within the delivery of health services by incorporating a case-control data collection process within established health information and surveillance systems.

11.2 DISASTERS

11.2.1 Introduction and Guidelines for Using the Case-Control Method in Disaster Investigation

Saylor and Gordon, in their 1957 classic review of the role of epidemiology in disasters (2), applied the concepts of epidemic investigation to disasters, recommending the use of epidemiologic approaches for solving problems in disaster situations. They proposed that a single impact disaster can be studied like a point epidemic, and in general the medical problems during the disaster can be studied along distributions of time, place, and persons.

There are a number of similarities in the investigation of outbreaks and the epidemiologic assessments of disasters. Beyond the fact that both disasters and outbreaks occur in acute or urgent circumstances, the following are some common guidelines for the epidemiologist who is faced with these situations:

- The epidemiologist needs to be trained and prepared well in advance to deal with these situations. When a disaster strikes there is very little time to plan a study or develop the instruments for the investigation, which could explain why most disasters have not been investigated by epidemiologists in the past.
- The epidemiologic investigation needs to be part and parcel of an information system that feeds into the decision-making process, aimed, first and foremost, at relieving the suffering of those affected by the disaster.
- The situation may have to be reassessed on an ongoing basis and some of the approaches and the content of the investigation may be modified with the changing circumstances. The decisions that need to be made may evolve as new issues about the management of the disaster are discovered.

Thus, in addition to providing a well-defined approach to disaster investigation, the use of some of the steps of outbreak investigation will help organize an approach as well as provide us with a framework for training in disaster epidemiology.

11.2.2 The 1988 Earthquake in Armenia, and Other Examples

The case-control method presents with major advantages of efficiency and informativeness in disaster situations. Within hours of the occurrence of the disaster, one may be able to design and implement a case-control investigation and provide the results of the analysis within a few days.

Thus, within weeks of the massive 1988 earthquake of Northern Armenia, a case-control study was set up to assess the determinants of hospitalized injuries as a result of the earthquake (3). The investigation was part of an evaluation of the health conditions in the survivors of the earthquake. The cases were persons who were hospitalized with injuries from Giumry, the largest city affected by the earthquake, and the site of over 60% of earthquake-related deaths. The controls were persons who had not been hospitalized for injuries as a result of the earthquake and were selected through lists available in the neighborhood polyclinics. Due to the destruction of many buildings and blocks, random sampling and identification of controls were not possible, even with the use of pre-earthquake maps. Exposure information included location of the individual at the moment of the earthquake, building or housing structural characteristics, pre-earthquake life styles and traits, actions immediately following the earthquake, family history, losses, and impact of the earthquake. The study identified protective behaviors during the disaster as well as building and structural factors that contributed to injury. Running out of the building at the first instance of the earthquake was protective for injuries, and being located in high rise structures represented a high risk.

A number of other case-control investigations in other disasters and earthquakes have been conducted since this study was published. The most difficult problems in these case-control studies are defining and identifying cases and controls and assessing exposure. Considering that these are population-wide disasters, almost everyone is exposed to some degree. Thus, the comparison of cases and controls need to focus on differences in the intensity of exposure rather than a dichotomous exposed versus nonexposed categorization. Daley and colleagues studied the risk of tornado-related deaths and severe injuries in a major disaster in Oklahoma in 1999 using the case-control approach (4). The cases were deaths and severe injuries, while the controls were individuals who were interviewed as part of a survey of the population in the damage path. The risk of death and severe injuries was greater for those who were in mobile homes or outdoors.

11.3 POTENTIAL APPLICATIONS OF CASE-CONTROL ANALYSIS IN DIFFERENTIAL MORTALITY STUDIES

11.3.1 Background

Studies of mortality differences across population subgroups, defined on the basis of characteristics that include socioeconomic status, educational level, and country of birth, are particularly fruitful for generating hypotheses about the sociodemographic factors underlying ill-health. National or subnational death rates are based on death registration data (numerator) and census tabulations (denominator), and a frequent difficulty concerns the degree of consistency between definitions of the classification factor on the death certificate and on the census form.

At best, the definitions are consistent, and the population at risk is based on intercensal estimates; at worst, that population is not known at all. The latter situation may arise when, for instance, data on the criterion of interest are recorded in civil registers and those of the census forms cannot be matched. The only figures available then are proportional mortality data consisting of numbers of deaths classified by age at death, cause of death, year of death, and other factors of interest.

11.3.2 Rationale of the Case-Control Analysis of Proportional Mortality Data

Under certain conditions, data of this type can be considered as arising from a case-control study, in which cases are deaths from the causes of interest, and controls are deaths from other causes, to be chosen appropriately. If we can reasonably assume those "controls" to be unrelated to the "exposure" under study, then the resulting odds ratios can be considered as good estimators of the relative risk of death from the cause of interest (5,6).

When investigating mortality from specific cancers, controls may be either (1) deaths from other cancers, (2) deaths from all other causes, or (3) deaths from all other causes excluding cancers. One method of evaluating the three groups as potential controls is to compare the estimates attached to each with those based on mortality rates, using a dataset comprising appropriate denominator figures (7). Estimates of risks of dying from several cancers for Italian migrants in Australia relative to Australian-born individuals were studied, and of the three "control groups," the one with associated estimates closest to those based on the mortality rates was the "other cancers" control group. More generally, this approach is well suited to the study of cancer mortality in migrants, and has been applied for this purpose.

11.3.3 Case Studies

11.3.3.1 *Death from melanoma in immigrants to Australia.*   In an investigation of the risk of death from melanoma in immigrants to Australia (8), the data comprised all deaths registered during the period 1964–1985, with information on state of registration of death, year of registration of death, sex, age at death, country of birth, duration of stay in Australia, year of death, and cause of death code. Population-at-risk data by age, sex, and country of birth were available from the censuses of 1966, 1971, 1976, and 1981. However, breakdown by state was not available for 1966 and 1971, and duration of stay was missing in 1976 for 36% of overseas-born, and was, in any case, only available for categories of irregular length, which changed with each census. For those reasons, interpolation of the population at risk was difficult, and analysis had to be restricted to numerator (death) data. Logistic regression models were fitted for the main groups of male immigrants originating from outside Oceania, considering deaths from other cancers as controls, with the findings shown in Table 11.1.

No significant difference in risk was found between male immigrants from England and immigrants from Ireland, Scotland, and Wales: in both groups, the risk remained below that of the Australian-born, with almost no change until 30 years of residence in Australia, and then an increase was evident. Immigrants from Central Europe experienced an increase in estimated risk with longer duration of stay, and the estimates for duration of 30 years or more do not differ significantly from the Australian-born. Among immigrants from Eastern Europe, the patterns were less clear, while Southern Europeans remained at lower estimated

Table 11.1. Estimated Relative Risks of Death from Melanoma by Duration of Stay in Australia Compared with the Australian-Born

Region of Birth	Duration of Stay in Australia (years)[a]			
	<10	10–19	20–29	30+
England	0.34 (0.23–0.49)	0.23 (0.16–0.33)	0.31 (0.22–0.44)	0.68 (0.58–0.79)
Ireland/Scotland/ Wales[b]	0.21 (0.10–0.48)	0.27 (0.16–0.46)	0.24 (0.13–0.43)	0.63 (0.50–0.79)
Central Europe	0.17 (0.04–0.69)	0.38 (0.23–0.64)	0.52 (0.37–0.73)	0.82 (0.55–1.22)
Eastern Europe	0.40 (0.15–1.08)	0.34 (0.19–0.60)	0.48 (0.33–0.69)	0.41 (0.27–0.61)
Southern Europe	0.22 (0.11–0.47)	0.21 (0.13–0.33)	0.31 (0.21–0.45)	0.45 (0.33–0.62)
Western Asia[c]	0.49 (0.21–1.11)	0.51 (0.24–1.10)	0.02 (0.00–0.78)	0.47 (0.17–1.26)
Eastern Asia	0.10 (0.02–0.38)	0.10 (0.01–0.72)	0.82 (0.38–1.76)	0.48 (0.18–1.29)

[a] 95% confidence interval in parentheses.
[b] includes Northern Ireland and the Republic of Ireland
[c] based on very small numbers.

Risks adjusted for age, period, cohort, and state of registration of death.

risks than the Australian-born throughout their lives in Australia, even though their risk increased with lengthening duration of stay. The estimates in immigrants from Western Asia were almost all lower than 1, but failed to reach statistical significance in most cases, due to the small sample size. Low-risk estimates were also found in immigrants from Eastern Asia, with a tendency toward higher estimated risks for longer durations of stay in Australia.

To investigate possible biases in using other cancers as controls, the investigators repeated the analysis with alternative control groups: other noncancer deaths and all deaths from other causes (i.e., including other cancers). The ordering of the migrant groups with respect to their estimated relative risk of death from melanoma and the overall patterns of the estimated relative risks by duration of stay remained essentially unchanged.

11.3.3.2 *Differential cancer mortality by education in São Paulo, Brazil.* The same methodology was adopted to examine differential cancer mortality by education in São Paulo, Brazil, where categorization of educational level in census forms and death certificates were not compatible (9). Differential cancer incidence by place of birth or ethnicity was also explored in the same way in populations where the appropriate denominator figures were not available (10,11).

11.3.4 Limitations

One limitation of the case-control analysis of proportional mortality data is that it can only be applied to investigate mortality differences with regard to specific causes of death, or groups of causes, since no controls can be defined if general mortality is of interest, as all deaths are then eligible as cases. The challenges of using dead controls or cancer controls have been extensively discussed from epidemiological (12,13) and statistical (14) perspectives, and it is clear that, depending on the causes chosen, real effects could be masked, or spurious effects could be generated. The main difficulty is therefore choosing appropriate controls: the implicit assumption when selecting as controls a mix of causes of death, other than the cause of interest is that any cause-specific biases will cancel each other out. This is also the reasoning behind the use of several admission categories in hospital-based case-control studies. Alternatively, the investigator could use several control groups in parallel, since the reproducibility of the results considerably reinforces the conclusions of this type of study.

11.4 OCCUPATIONAL STUDIES

11.4.1 Description and Challenges

The case-control method has been used in a number of occupational studies to identify various risk factors and assess results of interventions. Checkoway and Demers (15) in their review of such case-control studies identify three types of case-control studies in occupational epidemiology: (1) case-control studies nested within occupational cohorts; (2) community-based case-control studies using data from registries or similar sources; and (3) record linkage studies whereby disease information is collected from registries, and vital records and occupational data from other existing data sources such as employment information.

According to Siematicky and colleagues (16), properly conducted occupational case-control studies convey as much information as do cohort studies. They proposed a system whereby the case-control method is part of the ongoing surveillance and investigation program for occupational diseases as described in the first section of this chapter.

Issues of case identification and control selection in occupational epidemiology are similar to other epidemiological studies except that for a large number of these studies an occupational cohort is easier to identify if employment data are routinely collected by the industry. The presence of such data bases makes it possible to identify both the cases and the controls from the same cohort and conduct a nested case-control study.

The major challenge for the use of case-control studies in occupational epidemiology is the measurement of exposure. In the absence of well-kept employment and environmental exposure records it will be very difficult to collect such information from the individual cases and controls over several decades. Thus, much of the effort in these studies needs to focus on gathering valid exposure data. Stewart and colleagues (17) described a computer-assisted interview schedule that will collect as a routine a generic work history, as well as other relevant data in modular format, for potential nested case-control analyses in occupational cohorts.

11.4.2 Exposure to Pesticides and the Risk of Non-Hodgkin's Lymphoma in Australia

To investigate occupational exposure to pesticides and the risk of non-Hodgkin's lymphoma in Australia, Fritschi et al. conducted a population-based case-control study using detailed methods of assessing occupational pesticide exposure (18). Cases were incident non-Hodgkin's lymphomas from two states and controls were chosen from electoral rolls. "The major limitation of the exposure assessment method we used was its cost. Review of job histories, administration of telephone interviews, and review of responses to the assigned occupational modules are highly labor-intensive. In addition, lengthy consultation with experts in agriculture, farming, and pesticide exposure monitoring was required to construct the pesticide exposure matrix. Use of an existing job exposure matrix would have been less intensive but possibly subject to significant nondifferential misclassification" (p. 855). Substantial exposure to any pesticide was associated with an odds ratio of 3.09 (95% confidence interval: 1.42, 6.70) and none of the exposure metrics (probability, level, frequency, duration, or years of exposure) were associated with non-Hodgkin's lymphoma (18).

11.4.3 Occupational Risk Factors for Cancers among Female Textile Workers in Shanghai, China: a Case-Cohort Design

In two separate reports, the authors used the case-cohort design to link occupational exposures in the textile industry and the risks of esophageal, stomach, and liver cancers. In separate analyses they compared 102 incident cases of esophageal cancer, 646 incident cases of stomach cancer, and 360 liver cancer cases to the same comparison group of 3,188 age-stratified randomly chosen subcohort from a cohort of 267,400 female textile workers. Exposures to workplace dust and chemicals were reconstructed from work history data. They estimated relative risks and dose-response trends using Cox proportional hazards models, adapted for the case-cohort design. In addition to increased risk for cancer due to long-term exposure to silica and metals they observed a protective effect for exposure to endotoxin (19,20).

11.5 FUTURE APPLICATIONS

In this chapter and previous chapters a number of current and potential applications of the case-control method were illustrated. The method has come to age (21) over the past 50 years and is probably one of the most extensively used methods in epidemiology, medicine, and public health. We have seen a significant increase in both the breadth of its applications and the number of its users.

As to future developments, epidemiologists will continue innovating with newer applications of other case-based methods such the case-crossover and the case-cohort studies. Newer applications for these variants of the case-control method will be tested and potential problems to such applications identified.

The current explosion of information and its accompanying technologies make it possible to conduct case-control and other epidemiological studies much faster and in a timelier manner for decision making in public health and medicine. This will exponentially improve the efficiency of epidemiology as a problem-solving discipline for all concerned.

REFERENCES

1. Pasternack BS, Shore RE. Sample sizes for group sequential cohort and case-control study designs. *Am J Epidemiol*. 1981;113:182-191.
2. Saylor LF Gordon JE. The medical component of natural disasters. *Am J Med Sci*. 1957;234:342-362.
3. Armenian HK, Noji EK, Oganesian AP. A case-control study of injuries due to the earthquake in Armenia. *Bull WHO*. 1992;70:251-257.
4. Daley WR, Brown S, Archer P, et al. Risk of tornado-related death and injury in Oklahoma, May 3, 1999. Am J Epidemiol. 2005;161:1144-1150.
5. Khlat M. Use of case-control methods for indirect estimation in demography. *Epidemiol Rev*. 1994;16(1):124-133.
6. Kaldor J, Khlat M, Parkin DM, et al. Log-linear models for cancer risks among migrants. *Int J Epidemiol*. 1990;19:233-239.
7. Khlat M, Balzi D. Statistical methods. In: Geddes M, Parkin DM, Khlat M, et al., eds. *Cancer in Italian Migrant Populations*. Lyon, France: International Agency for Research on Cancer; 1993 (IARC Scientific Publication No. 123): 37-47.
8. Khlat M, Vail A, Parkin DM, et al. Mortality from melanoma in migrants to Australia: variation by age at arrival and duration of stay. *Am J Epidemiol*. 1992;135:1103-1113.
9. Bouchardy C, Parkin M, Khlat M, et al. Education and mortality from cancer in São Paulo, Brazil. *Ann Epidemiol*. 1993;3:64-70.
10. Bouchardy C, Mirra AM, Khlat M, et al. Ethnicity and cancer risk in São Paulo, Brazil. *Cancer Epidemiol Biomark Prev*. 1991;1:21-27.
11. Parkin M, Steinitz R, Khlat M, et al. Cancer in Jewish migrants to Israël. *Int J Cancer*. 1990;45:614-621.
12. Linet MS, Brookmeyer R. Use of cancer controls in case-control cancer studies. *Am J Epidemiol*. 1987;125:1-11.
13. Pearce N, Checkoway H. Case-control studies using other diseases as controls: problem of excluding exposure-related diseases. *Am J Epidemiol*. 1988;127:851-856.
14. Breslow NE, Day NE. *Statistical Methods in Cancer Research. Volume II. the Design and Analysis of Cohort Studies* (IARC Scientific Publication No. 82). Lyon: International Agency for Research on Cancer; 1987: 115-118.
15. Checkoway H, Demers PA. Occupational case-control studies. *Epidemiol Rev*. 1994;16:152-162.
16. Siematicky J, Day NE, Fabry J, Cooper JA. Discovering Carcinogens in the occupational environment: a novel epidemiologic approach. *JNCI*. 1981;66:217-225.

17. Stewart PA, Stewart WF, Heinman EF, Dosemeci M, Linet M, Inskip PD. A novel approach to data collection in a case-control study of cancer and occupational exposures. *Int J Epidemiol.* 1996; 25:744-752.
18. Fritschi L, Benke G, Hughes AM, et al. Occupational exposure to pesticides and risk of non-Hodgkin's lymphoma. *Am J Epidemiol.* 2005;162:849-857.
19. Wernli KJ, Fitzgibbons ED, Ray RM, et al. Occupational risk factors for esophageal and stomach cancers among female textile workers in Shanghai, China. *Am J Epidemiol.* 2006;163:717-725.
20. Chang CK, Astrakianis G, Thomas DB, et al. Occupational exposures and risks of liver cancer among Shanghai female textile workers – a case-control study. *Int J Epidemiol.* 2006;35:361-369.
21. Armenian HK, Gordis L. Future perspectives on the case-control method. *Epidemiol Rev.* 1994;16:163-164.

INDEX